DIABETES 2023
FROM FOLKLORE TO BIOTECHNOLOGY

AN EXPLORATION OF DIABETES AND MODERN INSULIN FOR THE GENERAL READER

S.K.Sinha

DIABETES 2023. FROM FOLKLORE TO BIOTECHNOLOGY
An Exploration of Diabetes and Insulin for the general reader

S K Sinha

ISBN: 978-0-6489470-4-2 (paperback)
ISBN: 978-0-6489470-5-9 (eBook)

© Copyright: S K Sinha 2024

Cover Design and typesetting by Publicious Book Publishing
Cover image: Above The Vines, Meursault, France.
Acrylic on canvas. 75 cm x 50 cm. by Lee Sinha ©

Published with the assistance of Publicious Book Publishing
www.publicious.com.au

To my wife Lee.

Pitaji Sukhdeo Sinha (1907–1961), my father.

Bhaiya Abhai Sinha (1929–2022), my brother
who sent me to medical school.

Also by S.K.Sinha

100 Years Of Insulin.

Joslin A Pioneer in Diabetes Care.

A Doctor's Wisdom For Diabetics.

The Sayings of Elliott Proctor Joslin.

Translation (Hindi to English)

Savera (The Morning) by J.S.Kanwal.

Contents

Introduction

"Tell the old story for our modern times."

Homer: The Odyssey. (7th century BCE)

*The history of medicine is the history of life and death,
and we are all connected to it.*

Mission Statement.

The Royal College of Physicians, England. Founded by King Henry VIII in 1518.

This book describes the journey of diabetes, one of the oldest ailments in human history. In Sanskrit there are over 30 definitions of journey but perhaps more useful are the terms used in old French and Vulgar (Colloquial) Latin. In Old French, *journee*, now obsolete, refers to work or to a day's travel. In colloquial Latin a *journeyer* is a traveller.

The journey of diabetes began in the time of the pharaohs and seers who believed that diseases and other misfortunes which plagued mankind were carried in the air. *Miasma*, a word derived from ancient Greek for pollution was the theory advanced by Hippocrates in the fourth century and held sway throughout the ancient world including Europe and China until the late 1800s when it was replaced by the "germ" theory. As late as the 1850s, cholera in London and in Paris was explained as a manifestation of miasma.

As recently as early 19th century some still believed that inhaling unsuitable air caused many ailments including obesity.

Diabetes also has a history of escaping scrutiny. It fails to make the lists of "old diseases." These are dominated by infectious diseases such as the bubonic plague, leprosy, tuberculosis, malaria and smallpox. Their prominence in recorded history lies in the accounts of epidemics.

The early descriptions of diabetes were chronicled in Egyptian hieroglyphics from the time of the pharaohs.

During the years of darkness when it's nature was a mystery and defied all attempts at unlocking its secrets, diabetes persisted in the myths and legends of many cultures and countries.

As agrarian life displaced the earlier hunter-gatherer existence of mankind, human beings became vulnerable to epidemics of infectious diseases. By and large, these were controlled or eradicated by the use of antibiotics, improved sanitation and immunisation. Books on the bubonic plague and other epidemics can be found in modern libraries in the history section.

Diabetes of epidemic proportions bided its time before coming to the fore as is recounted in this work.

Diabetes is invisible. There is nothing obvious which would distinguish such an individual from any other member of the community. Yet it's treatment requires daily attention, frequently more than once each 24 hours.

Today millions of men, women and children suffer from diabetes. The adults with the condition play their roles in society without bringing to the attention of their fellow workers the different lives they lead compared to those who are not affected. In fact throughout my years of treating these men, women and children I did not come across one who wanted to complain about his or her condition to others.

Nor are the elderly spared. The needs of the senior citizens represent special challenges for those involved in their care. Here the expertise of geriatricians makes their inclusion in the team caring for the elderly with diabetes, invaluable.

Long before it's discovery physicians had suspected that an element within the body played an important role in causing diabetes. Their convictions were strong enough to name that elusive substance insuline.

Insulin holds a unique position in medical history. It's discovery ranks as one of the most significant events in medical research. The successful identification and isolation of insulin in 1921 changed the lives of millions around the world.

To say that the discovery was greeted with euphoria would be an understatement. Before insulin, children who had diabetes often did not live longer than 3 to 4 years. Even a minor illness like influenza meant possible loss of life. The burden of fear and apprehension borne by their parents was common knowledge. Little wonder then that stories of courage shown by children and young people with diabetes as well as the unspoken sacrifices made by their parents have entered the annals of medical folklore.

The use of insulin in the treatment of those who suffer from diabetes is rightly celebrated as "a daily miracle."

Insulin transformed their future from the possibility of an early death to the reality of fruitful lives. They could marry, have families, pursue ambitions, gain higher education and as adults, make contributions to society in numerous ways, including spectacular accomplishments, which in turn improved the lot of their fellow human beings.

Those who need insulin need to check the level of glucose in the blood before giving themselves one or more injections every day.

For them insulin is indeed a daily miracle.

Little wonder then that following its discovery the hormone became an intensive focus of medical and laboratory research. Remarkable advances followed including further insights into the chemical make-up of insulin. Newly developed instruments of investigation, including crystallography and electron microscopy were employed, revealing further insights into the biological nature of cells and organs which were being studied by scientists in a wide range of disciplines. In diabetes the improvements in the different preparations of insulin overcame many of the disadvantages such as allergic reactions, which troubled patients from the use of the original form.

The worldwide community of physicians and scientists continues to work on this particular aspect of the treatment of this condition.

Continuing research in modern times also underlies many recent discoveries into the nature of insulin which is detailed in this work.

In the second half of the 20th century, a spectacular leap of scientific accomplishment heralded a remarkable advance in the treatment of diabetes with "modern" insulin which no longer has to rely on supplies of animal pancreases.

Newer technologies have now enabled individuals with diabetes to measure blood sugar levels through sensing devices without resorting to finger pricks. Similarly, automatic delivery systems for insulin using indwelling fine plastic tubes (catheters) are examples of the giant strides made in the treatment of insulin-requiring diabetes through medical research.

The search for insulin in 1920 was the journey of a lone medical graduate largely unversed in medical research.

How different were his experiences from those whose accomplishments adorn the story of the development of modern insulin.

Unlike Banting who, except for his one student-helper, was a lone researcher in search of insulin, the team which developed modern insulin features a dizzying array of academic talent including Nobel laureates, professors and "graduate students" who already had doctorates in different branches of science. Although driven by an insatiable thirst to discover "the inner workings" of cells in the human body, they were not narrow in their approach to life. For example, one was a fearless rock climber, another a university professor who marched in every anti-war rally held in San Francisco in the post-Vietnam era. And how could I possibly leave out the gold medal winning medical student who also played the 5-string banjo and the ukulele and composed songs, one which made it into the "hit parade". He later became a respected professor who played a critical role in the development of modern insulin.

The story of insulin is a journey in itself. It is a journey within the journey of diabetes. In this account, insulin's journey is described separately after the journey of diabetes.

The discovery which produced what I refer to as "modern insulin" was the main reason for undertaking this project.

This work is intended for the general reader. I have minimised the use of technical terms and expressions and have written as I would to a friend interested in, but not familiar with, diabetes.

Over the years, Boileau's maxim has kept me from straying into medical jargon.

Ce qui ce concoit clairement, S'expresse clairement.
That which one understands clearly, One can express clearly.

First, the answers to two frequently-asked questions on diabetes.

What is Diabetes?

Central to the understanding of diabetes is the role of a hormone called insulin which is made in the pancreas, a 6-inch long, comma-shaped organ which sits behind the stomach and intestines.

A lack of, or insufficient insulin is the chief cause of diabetes in young people. Therefore, a daily supply of insulin together with a diet restricted in sugar is the most important part of treatment. This form of diabetes is usually called Type 1 diabetes. its treatment requires the use of insulin.

It differs from diabetes in middle-aged and older adults in whom it is referred to as Type 2 or Adult Onset diabetes. Unlike Type 1 diabetes, the adult form is often controlled with tablets, which together with a diet can often control the condition satisfactorily.

In Type 2 diabetes insulin is often present in higher than normal amounts because the body is resistant to its effect. Such individuals are often referred to as being "insulin resistant" and their diabetes is called Type 2 or Insulin Resistant Diabetes.

The two types of diabetes may well be described as conditions caused by *insufficient insulin,* in Type 1 and *inefficient insulin* in Type 2 diabetes.

Secondly, why is the dose of insulin measured in units?

The amount of insulin needed is different for every individual with diabetes. It is measured in "units". One unit of insulin is a standardised amount which is employed in all countries where insulin is used for treating diabetes.

One unit of insulin is the amount of the hormone, which will lower the level of blood glucose by a standard amount. It is the amount of insulin required to lower the blood glucose of a rabbit by 2.5 mmol per litre. This was established shortly after the discovery of insulin in Toronto, Canada in 1921.

We now know that one unit of insulin by weight is 0.0347 mg of crystalline insulin. Little wonder that the original way of measuring insulin in units is still in use. It would be a nightmare to measure insulin by weight for each patient.

Diabetes "The Three Ps Condition".

The three Ps are *polyuria*, *polydipsia* and *polyphagia*. Polyphagia is a feeling of constant hunger which leads an individual to eat more than is needed by the body.

A basic problem in diabetes is that the body is not able to convert the glucose obtained from the food consumed into energy. This causes the glucose level in the blood to rise higher than is normal. An abnormally high blood glucose level is often the first sign of diabetes which is detected by a blood test.

The abnormally high levels of sugar (glucose) in the blood make the kidneys produce more urine so as to remove the excess glucose from the body.

Together with glucose, the body also loses fluids. This leads to the two commonest complaints in diabetes – the patient has to pass urine more frequently, *polyuria* in medical jargon, and second, because the body is losing fluids through frequent passage of urine, the patient becomes uncontrollably thirsty and drinks more water, *polydipsia*.

Therefore, the story of diabetes is the story of a journey starting in the obscurity of ancient history and continuing in the 21st-century.

Equally intriguing is the account of insulin which the body needs to combat diabetes. The insulin narrative is presented as another journey. Insulin which was at first elusive, then obscure, turned out to be perhaps the brightest star in the new constellation of discoveries. The insulin journey introduces us to scientists and researchers from many countries who possess that rare combination of acute perception, stamina, and the never-say-die attitude which has provided remarkable benefits for men, women and children with diabetes.

Then fast-forward to early 20th century when we witness the drama of the discovery of insulin by a young Canadian doctor with limited experience in medical research.

The discovery which is often ranked as the most remarkable in human history brought about miraculous transformations in the lives of children and adults with diabetes.

Although earlier workers in the field did not have the advantages of technology as is the case today, what comes across is how prescient the earlier physicians and scientists were when their theories were little more than speculations. They battled lack of technology with sheer hard work and perseverance.

This work also describes how the "new" insulin was developed in the second half of the 20th century through breathtaking scientific advances on several fronts culminating in the production of "modern" insulin. Whereas in former times insulin was made from beasts, the new insulin is made from bacteria, "germs," we used to call them.

Today, between eight and nine million individuals around the world use insulin to control their diabetes. Once considered an affliction of the affluent, diabetes is now challenging the entire human race.

When caring for children with diabetes, one or both parents, attend to these and other related daily tasks seven days a week, 365 days a year, every year until the young are able to care for themselves.

The journeys of diabetes and of insulin are treated separately in this work.

The stories of some of the remarkable men and women who have made significant contributions to both these journeys are woven into the fabric of this account.

Stories of famous men and women with diabetes are presented to support the well recognised fact that diabetes is no barrier to accomplishments in virtually any field of human endeavour, including science and sport.

The stories and contributions of teachers and mentors of the younger scientists, researchers and physicians are included to honour them.

History has forgotten some of these men and women.

A Personal Note: My Mentors.

I was mentored by two men in the early years of my postgraduate studies.

Dr. Len Fienberg (1928–2020), was a remarkable man who for much of his professional life was in medical administration as the CEO of Ryde Hospital where I worked. A respected and highly qualified obstetrician-gynaecologist, Len was a graduate of Sydney University. After completing his early training in Sydney, he worked as a ship's doctor to travel to Britain where he gained postgraduate qualifications in Obstetrics and Gynaecology from the Royal Colleges of London and Edinburgh.

His support and guidance throughout my years in consultant practice were invaluable to me.

One incident which was typical of Len's thoughtfulness happened when shortly after my return to Sydney from the United States he sensed that I had limited funds to look after a young family. "I can lend you $7000 to buy a car. Try to avoid getting into debt," he said.

Len helped many young doctors especially those who had migrated to Australia from countries which were liberated after the fall of Communism.

Even after our professional association had ended with his retirement, we often met for lunch. He liked to speak of his interest in modern music especially jazz. Len died in 2020, a few months short of 93.

James Isbister Sr. (1915-1996), one of the leading physicians in Sydney, was the Senior Consultant Physician at The Royal North Shore Hospital in Sydney. His father, also called James, but better known through his initials "JLT" had been a prominent Obstetrician and Gynaecologist in Sydney. He had met William Osler, regarded by many as the father of modern medicine.

James was one of my tutors when I was a student. After graduation I had worked in his unit as an intern and later as his registrar.

During my time at the Joslin Clinic in Boston for postgraduate studies in diabetes, my wife and I were surprised and deeply moved by James's visit to us. His help and guidance especially in the early years of my practice in Sydney were invaluable and our friendship continued throughout his life. I was fortunate to keep in touch with James when he moved away from Sydney during the final years of his retirement.

The help and influence of such men is part of the history of the professional lives of many younger graduates. The stories of some of the mentors and teachers and their contributions to diabetes are described in different sections of this book.

That diabetes continues to defy elucidation of some of the underlying mechanisms responsible for its many effects on the human body guarantees that it will remain at the forefront not only of the scientific community but also governments, industries and private enterprise, all of whom are stakeholders with their interests ranging from the personal to the social and governmental.

Part One

Mysterious Journeys

1

ON THE BANKS OF THE NILE
WITH PHARAOHS

"What matters in life is not what happens to you, but how you remember it."

Gabriel Garcia Marquez.

The Egyptians did not have a name for the Nile. They simply called it *Iteru*, the river.

According to the Greek historian Herodotus, the southern part of the country, Lower Egypt, was "a gift of the river" which nourished the Sahara desert and enabled the natives to develop one of the earliest civilisations.

The Nile is arguably the longest river in the world. From its source in north-eastern Africa, it flows over 6600 km (just over 4000 miles), before reaching the Mediterranean Sea.

According to most authorities, the Egyptian civilisation, dated between 3100BC to 30 BC, was pre-dated only by the civilisation of Mesopotamia which existed between 3500 BC and 500 BC.

At that time, diabetes was thought to be caused by breathing in air which bore unspecified noxious agents, the so-called miasma theory. The treatment of the condition at this stage included mixtures of elderberry, plant fibres, beer, milk, flowers and green dates. It is thought- provoking that as recently as the beginning of the 20th century diabetes was essentially a disorder with no specific treatment.

Both the Mesopotamians and the Egyptians had developed writing. The Mesopotamians had invented writing, a cuneiform script but the first writings on diabetes were in Egyptian hieroglyphics. They were found in the Egyptian papyrus and were brought to the notice of the modern world by the German Egyptologist, George Ebers in the early 1870s. The Ebers Papyrus documented the ancient history of Egyptian medical knowledge in the time of the pharaohs dating back to 1550 BC.

Other papyri have been discovered, but Ebers' remains one of the oldest preserved records. It is kept in the University library of Leipzig in Germany.

Medical knowledge including the treatment of diabetes recorded in the papyrus included concoctions of fruit such as elderberry and dates as well as vegetables including cucumber, milk and beer-swill together with the as yet unidentified, "asit plant fibres".

In ancient times it was believed that the condition was visited upon hapless mankind by divine decree and spread through inhaling polluted vapours. This so-called *miasma theory* as the cause of many diseases including diabetes was preached and promulgated by seers, preachers and pundits in the eastern as well as western civilisations.

The actual beginnings of diabetes are are still shrouded in the mists of antiquity with no clear indication of just when it was first recognised as an affliction of mankind. At that time there was scant knowledge of the nature of normal bodily characteristics, let alone details of disease. Studies of basic bodily characteristics through branches of learning, including anatomy, and physiology were not known. Neither did early man have the tools to help in investigating abnormal conditions. Pathology as a branch of learning was described in the history of medicine many years later.

The earliest mention of diabetes in recorded history is found in the time of the pharaohs of Egypt as described above.

It is a challenging mental exercise to reconcile the remarkable achievements and sophistication in the lives and times of the ancient Egyptian pharaohs with the fact that they existed more than 3000 years ago. Their stories are part of an astounding and fascinating civilisation in the dawn of human history.

In recent years, the pharaoh Tutankhamun has become the subject of interest largely because of the discovery of his tomb in 1922, which was intact. Other tombs in the Valley of the Kings, many of which had been discovered earlier, had been plundered.

However, the history of insulin began hundreds of years earlier than the reign of Tutankhamun which is dated from 1332 to 1323BC.

It was during the reign of the pharaoh Djoser dating back to a period between 2686 BC and 2648 BC, that we find history's oldest link to diabetes. It is of interest to begin the story of the Pharaohs with a brief description of the most prominent relic of their times as the rulers of Egypt.

The First Pyramid.

The pyramid of Djoser, built in the 27th century BC and named after the pharaoh buried within its confines, is said to be the oldest pyramid. Its modern location is in Egypt. Remarkably, this construction has, to a large extent, defied natural disasters and the passage of time. Following repairs and restorations carried out in the early 2000s, Djoser's pyramid was re-opened for visitors in 2020.

The Djoser pyramid introduces a charismatic individual to the ancient history of diabetes. The Wikipedia summary of the "Pyramid of Djoser" contains a single word as the name of the architect.

Imhotep.

Important as his construction is, there was more – much more – to Imhotep than designing the first pyramid.

Some consider him to be the first physician known by name in the written history of the world.

In later years, men with proficiency in several fields were referred to as "polymaths". Imhotep would certainly qualify for inclusion in this category of scholars.

In addition to architecture, he advised the Pharaoh on matters ranging from simple carpentry to the weather. He was also a seer.

Imhotep is the earliest named physician in ancient Egypt. He served the pharaoh Djoser who reigned from 2667–2648, BC.

The seer's main contribution from the point of view of this book is as the founder of Egyptian medicine and the author of the Smith and Ebers papyrus which contained references to diabetes. He also furnished information on collections of clinical records of medical specimens and clinical features of various injuries.

For his "invention" of healing Imhotep, soon after his death, was worshipped as a demigod.

In Greco–Roman times Imhotep was deified by the Greeks as the god of medicine, Asclepius.

Even in modern times, 2000 years later, in the Egyptian and Greek cultures Imhotep is considered a God of medicine and healing.

The Ebers Papyrus was said to be found between the legs of a mummy in the Theban Necropolis, which is a cemetery on the West Bank of the Nile, opposite Thebes in upper Egypt, and houses the tombs of pharaohs and nobles of Egypt. It includes the Valley of the Kings mentioned in the Bible as well as in the Jewish religious texts.

Originally purchased in Luxor by Edwin Smith in 1862, the material was sold to George Ebers, a German Egyptologist in 1872. Ebers published a facsimile in English and Latin three years later.

This, according to most authorities, is believed to be the oldest medical document and is dated from 1552 BC. After noting that more than 700 magical formulae, including incantations and folk remedies, which were described in the papyrus, the writers stated :

"Of great interest to endocrinologists is the opinion that in the Ebers Papyrus is the first known medical reference to diabetes mellitus. The comment refers to a single phrase which describes diabetes as a condition in which the individual suffering from it tries "… to eliminate urine, which is too plentiful."

There was also mention of excessive thirst. The treatment used was based on extracts of plants.

There has been a suggestion that some of the information contained in the papyrus maybe inaccurate. This is based on the opinion of the medical historian and Egyptian endocrinologist Paul Ghalioungui (1908–1987) who translated the Ebers papyrus.

Ghalioungui quoted information from the Kahun papyrus (circa 2000 BC), noting that there was a title of a recipe for "treatment of a thirsty woman" but the accompanying text was missing. Based on this, he suggested that ancient Egyptians may not have made the connection between disease states such as diabetes and complaints such as excessive thirst.

There are minor differences between the account described above and the article by William Rostene and Pierre DeMeyts: *Insulin: a Hundred Year-old Discovery With a Fascinating History* published in 2021 by Oxford University Press on behalf of the Endocrine Society.

According to this account the date of the discovery of the oldest manuscript was 1550 BC. It was found in a sarcophagus in Luxor and sold to Georg Moritz Ebers in 1872. The papyrus is now housed in the Leipzig University library.

A word on Georg Ebers (1837–1898).

Ebers came from a wealthy German family which was known for manufacturing porcelain. Georg Ebers however, chose an academic career and went to university where he studied Egyptology, a subject on which in later years he became a respected authority. Georg Ebers had come from a family of porcelain manufacturers. He owned a villa in Tutzing, a village on the shores of Lake Starnberg which is situated near Munich. Ebers had lived there in the latter part of his life. He died in 1898 and is buried in the Northern Cemetery in Munich.

The information on Ebers comes from a friend and colleague from the days of my Fellowship at the Joslin Clinic in Boston.

Professor Eberhard Standl, a third-generation physician, comes from a family which has been prominent in Munich for several generations.

Eberhard's father, Dr Rudolph Erich Standl (1912–2005), whom I met on more than one occasion, was a remarkable individual. Dr Rudolph Standl's father, also called Rudolph, was the Chief of Internal Medicine at Saint Elizabeth Hospital in Dorsten.

Professor Hellmut Mehnert (1928–2023), the Chief of Medicine and a friend and mentor of Eberhard Standl had been helped by Eberhard's father on his (Mehnert's) arrival in Munich as a recent medical graduate from the former East Germany.

Eberhard, who remains active in clinical and investigative medicine is one of the most sought-after lecturers on diabetes in conferences around the world.

Although by nature he is disinclined to speak of his many accomplishments, Eberhard has also been an accomplished athlete. Between 1982 and 1991 he ran nine full marathons, eight on the Munich marathon track (the original Olympic track of 1972) as well as the New York marathon in 1991.

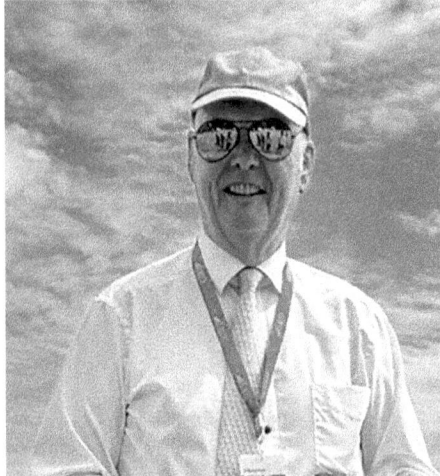

Professor Eberhard Standl.

2

A ROMAN EMPEROR IN A DOCTOR'S WAITING ROOM

Constantine, also known as Constantine the Great (272–337, A.D.) was the Roman emperor who ruled between 306–337 A.D. When he came to the throne, Rome was the capital of the Empire. Constantine decided to move the capital to Byzantium which became known as Constantinople after the Emperor which was later changed to the current name, Istanbul. When Constantine became the Emperor, the majority of physicians practised in Rome because of the prestige of the city. The Emperor set about persuading prominent physicians to move to the recently established city.

One of the most prominent physicians of that period was called Aretaeus who was born in Cappadocia, an area which today would occupy a position in the centre of Turkey. At that time Rome was the ruling power of Greek Asia Minor. Aretaeus had studied in Alexandria and practised there as well as in Rome.

There is no information on any prior contact between the Emperor and the physician. However, there was no likelihood of any citizen, no matter how prominent, acting against the wishes of the ruler. Furthermore, Constantine promised Aretaeus various rewards including the cost of moving his practice, as well as providing a suitable location and a home befitting a man renowned for his learning and expertise.

Although highly respected and much sought after for his wise counsel which he based on thorough observation, Aretaeus, the Cappadocian was not well known until his works were translated into Latin and published in Venice 1552.

From the point of view of diabetes this physician and scholar was one of the most knowledgeable, and his writings discovered many years after his death remain one of the most quoted whenever the topic of the early knowledge of diabetes is discussed.

3

A PHYSICIAN IN CONSTANTINOPLE. ARETAEUS OF CAPPADOCIA

"No medical author of antiquity surpasses Aretaeus in his vivid portrayal of disease."

Konstantinos Laios.

The earliest description of diabetes is attributed to Aretaeus, a famous physician who lived in the 2nd century AD.

According to the information found in medical publications written by Konstantinos Laois in Novo Scriptorium Aretaeus occupies a prestigious position amongst the physicians of that era and is considered second only to Hippocrates and equal to the Greek physician Galen.

The reasons for the writings of the respected Cappadocian not being translated into Latin until 1554 were not known until it was discovered that his manuscripts had been mislaid and not discovered till 1554, when two of the manuscripts *On the Causes and Indications of Acute and Chronic Diseases* (4 volumes), and *On the Treatment of Acute and Chronic disease* (4 volumes) were discovered. However, when the manuscripts were discovered, it was realised that Aretaeus wrote in the ionic Greek dialect. Hence the translation of the original works to Latin.

The translated versions were released in Venice in late 1554.

The second chapter of his second book was headed "On the Causes and Symptoms of Acute and Chronic Disease." It contains a clear description of several features of diabetes.

By contrast, there is no description of diabetes in the writings of Hippocrates.

As described above, Aretaeus' descriptions were contained in the Ebers Papyrus circa 1550 BC which were discovered in 1872 at Luxor by George Ebers, a German Egyptologist originally from Munich in Germany.

The Cappadocian and his contemporaries belonged to the so-called Eclectic School of Medicine because they respected previous publications on various medical conditions and tried to distinguish between the studies and practices based on sound and rational medical principles as opposed to unproven practices which in earlier times had carried over from long held beliefs and superstition.

However, Aretaeus was not entirely free of the medical beliefs at that time which included the role of the elements of nature in causing disease including diabetes. The Pneumatic School founded in the first century AD was based on the belief of that disease was caused by air and the four elements (humours), namely, heat, cold, moisture, and dryness. The adherence of this school maintained that health depended on "vital air" or *pneuma*. Remember, the previously held traditional belief was that disease was caused by mysterious substances carried by air together with an imbalance of the four humours, namely, blood, phlegm, yellow bile (choler) and melancholy (black bile). This imbalance disturbed the *pneuma*, a condition which they held was indicated by an abnormal pulse.

Therefore, the description of diabetes, as described below, includes the belief in the contribution of natural elements in the atmosphere having a role in causing diabetes.

This belief that disease was caused by unknown agents in the air was still held in the late 1800s and early 1900s and included respected scientists like the famous French chemist and microbiologist, Louis Pasteur (1822–1895), even though he (Pasteur) had discovered vaccination.

The eight volume treatise produced by the Greek physician is impressive not only for the amount of medical information it contains but also for the logical and systematic way that he deals with the medical subjects he describes.

This is seen in what is believed to be the first detailed description of diabetes.

Aretaeus systematically described diabetes more thoroughly than is found in many of the textbooks of General Medicine used in medical schools today.

He began with a description of the common complaints of patients with diabetes before proceeding to the cause/s of the condition which he believed included atmospheric factors such as a cold and humid atmosphere. The roles of the kidneys and bladder were emphasised as was "the melting" of the flesh. This last feature was considered to be responsible for the weight loss which is a characteristic of diabetes especially in younger patients.

Next the Cappadocian described the progression of the disease, which today's medical jargon is the "natural history" of diabetes.

Also included in his writings are descriptions of different causes of diabetes. Here Aretaeus engages in possible alternative explanations for the complaints in diabetes. In today's terminology this would be called the "differential diagnosis" of diabetes, a feature which was unusual, if not unique, in medical dissertations at that time.

Physicians and medical scholars were rightly stunned by the brilliance of the Cappadocian.

The thoroughness of his observations and the depth of his knowledge coupled with a gifted writing style provided the first lucid description of diabetes.

At that time the knowledge of diabetes was limited and descriptions of the condition were at best fragmentary. Physicians including Galen were the only medical sources of ancient Greek literature. Unfortunately, the Latin translation of much of this material has been lost.

"Diabetes uses man's body as a ladder," said Aretaeus to explain the passing of large quantities of urine. He called diabetes "a remarkable affliction"and pointed to the kidneys and bladder as the seat of the condition, because "the patients never stop making water, but the flow is incessant, as if from the opening of aqueducts…"

"The nature of the disease, then, is chronic, and it takes a long time to form; but the patient is short-lived if the constitution of the disease be completely established; for the melting is rapid, the death speedy."

Aretaeus then digressed to explain the reason for the disease being called diabetes, saying "the disease appears to me to have got the name diabetes as if from a Greek word which signifies a siphon, because the food does not remain in the body, but uses the man's body as a ladder whereby to leave it.

The Greek physician Galen is generally credited with having called the condition, diabetes. However, Galen himself had seen only two patients with the condition. The fact that diabetes is now a worldwide epidemic supports the view that it may be consequence of affluence.

The Cappadocian's vivid description of diabetes is worth quoting:

> *"Moreover, life is disgusting and painful; thirst, unquenchable; excessive drinking which however, is disproportionate to the large quantity of urine, for more urine is passed ; and one cannot stop them, either from drinking or making water.*
>
> *… if for a time they abstain from drinking, their mouth becomes parched and their body dry; the viscera seem as if scorched up; they are affected with nausea, restlessness, and a burning thirst; and at no distant term, they expire. They thirst, as if scorched up with fire…. but if it increases still more, the heat is small, indeed, but pungent, and seated in the intestine's; the abdomen*

is shrivelled, the veins protuberant, and there is general inanition, when the quantity of urine in the first have already increased; and when, at the same time, the sensation of burning of the extremity of the member, the patients immediately make water. hence the disease appears to me to have got the name diabetes is it from the Greek word, which signifies a siphon, because the fluid does not remain in the body, what uses the man's body is a ladder whereby to leave it. They survive not for long and ……. many parts of the flesh passed out along with the urine."

The intensity of thirst in diabetes defies description.

I was told about this on several occasions by patients who spoke of the thirst they had experienced before starting their treatment. The need to quench their thirst often led to desperate measures to find drinking water. One patient was arrested in a public toilet by the city police who claimed they had caught him damaging public property when someone had seen him climb onto the seat of the toilet to reach up to the tank which, in the models in use in the 1970s, held water for flushing after use. He was taken to the local court but fortunately released when he told the magistrate of his diabetes.

Another experience which echoes the desperate plight of an individual with diabetes needing to quench his thirst is that of a group of travellers stranded in a desert when their supplies of water had run out.

There is a graphic description of the incident in William Atkins's *The Immeasurable World. A Desert Journey* (Faber and Faber, 2018).

The account is based on records held in a collection in the Royal Geographical Society (RGS) in London, England on the travels of the Swedish explorer, Sven Hedin in the Taklamakan desert in 1901. Hedin described the plight of some members of his party when, possibly through a miscalculation on his part, they ran out of water in the middle of the desert.

"His retinue tried to slake their thirst with camel's piss flavoured with vinegar and sugar, but were soon doubled up with nausea…

…Gaunt and wild eyed, with the stamp of insanity upon him, *Yolchi sat beside the tent, gnawing at the dripping sheep's lungs.

"Water, sir! Only a drop of water!" *Yolchi had pleaded.

Finally Hedin departed leaving Yolchi and *Mohammad Shah, both members of his party, to die,.

(* members of Hedon's party).

4

WRITINGS OF THE "CHINESE HIPPOCRATES" AND INDIAN SCHOLARS.

In the 5th century BC the renowned Indian surgeon Sushruta described some features of diabetes in his own writings titled *Samhita*. He gave the condition an Indian name *madhumeha* meaning honey urine. The description included an observation of the sweet taste of urine from a patient with diabetes as well as the specimen being sticky to touch and attracting ants to the specimen he had collected.

A blunt comment by the Indian surgeon was that the commonest cause of diabetes was excessive food intake by the wealthy individuals of the Hindu higher castes namely *Brahmins* and *Kshatriyas*. (I tried, unsuccessfully, to find Susruta's caste).

"The Chinese Hippocrates".

In circa 160 - circa 219, Chang Chung-Ching referred to by some as the Chinese Hippocrates, described polyuria, polydipsia and weight loss as the symptoms of a particular condition.

In the 7th century A.D. The Chinese physician, Chen Chuan documented that the urine of a patient was sweet and called the condition *Hsiao kho ping* meaning, sweet urine. He also described the common complaints of pronounced thirst, intake of large volume of liquids, and passage of copious amounts of urine. The treatment advised was abstinence from wine, salt, and sexual activity.

In this day and age of specialists and sub- specialists in many branches of medicine, it is of interest that the papyrus noted the comments of the Greek philosopher Herodotus on Egyptians that "medicine is practised among them on the plan of separation: each physician treats a single disease, and not more; thus the country abounds with physicians..."

Now in some countries, including the United States, doctors practising in narrow fields of medicine are referred to as "sub-specialists", or "super specialists". there is also a proliferation of new terms for different specialists. For example, a physician with subspecialty training in diabetes after specialising in Internal Medicine is referred to as a diabetologist.

From the eighth century onwards different physicians described various characteristics of diabetes such as skin infections including boils (furuncles) and deep ulcers. Poor eyesight was also noted but the details of this are vague.

5

ARABIAN BRILLIANCE. AVICENNA (980-1037 AD)

Avicenna is the Latin version of the name of an eminent Arab physician, whose real name was Abu Ali Al-Hussein ibn (meaning, son of) Abdullah Ibn Sina. He was born in 980 A.D. near the city of Bukhara in Central Asia which at the time was the capital of the Samani kingdom and is part of Uzbekistan today.

Considered a childhood prodigy, Avicenna had memorised the Quran by the age of 10 and was proficient in the Arabic language and it's classics. He embarked on studies in medicine at the age of 13 and completed the studies at the age of 18 by which time he was considered a well-established physician. His reputation extended well beyond Central Asia. As a reward for his successful treatment of the Sultan of Bukhara, Avicenna was given access to the royal library. Avicenna wrote a book on medicine and later moved to a town near the modern Tehran to practise medicine.

It is said that he had written some 450 documents of which 240 had survived, but there is disagreement over the actual number of his major or minor works which include philosophy, medicine, geometry and astronomy as well as topics on religion, philosophy, and art.

Avicenna's Writings on Medicine and Diabetes.

Avicenna's Canon on medicine is considered the most influential medical writing by a Muslim physician. It is a one million word document, containing the essentials of Arabian medicine including its Greek roots which were altered or modified by the personal observations of Avicenna. Significantly, this book was the textbook for medical education in Europe from the 12th to the 17th century and had been translated into Latin. The Latin version went through more than a dozen editions. There was also an edition in Hebrew.

Avicenna's descriptions of diabetes are significant in that they include two complications of the condition which are a challenge in the treatment of the complications of diabetes even in today's patients suffering from diabetes of long duration. They are gangrene and a decline of sexual functions. The Arab physician also described an abnormal increase in appetite and the passing of "sweet urine". Avicenna died in 1037 AD aged 57.

According to information contained in documents and textbooks available in the last hundred years, further scrutiny of diabetes appears to have ceased at the stage when the understanding of the condition was mostly centred on the profound thirst and the sweet taste of urine. It therefore followed that diabetes was the result of one or more as yet undiscovered or undefined abnormalities of the kidneys.

At this point in the history of diabetes, there is a period of around 700 years, when historians have failed to find any significant progress in understanding the condition. These are often referred to as "the dark years" or "the long eclipse."

6

THE MYSTERY OF THE MISSING DOCUMENTS ON DIABETES THE DEAD SEA SCROLLS, A POSSIBLE CLUE ?

The early descriptions of diabetes as described above were not included in textbooks written in English-speaking countries. For example the 13th and the 14th editions of Joslin's Diabetes Mellitus published in 1994 and 2005 respectively record a period exceeding some 1500 years when there was little if any progress on the condition. In fact, there is an absence of any references to diabetes in the timeline of the condition in medical textbooks in the period between 150 AD when the condition had been described by Aretaeus to the second half of the 17th century when the English physician Thomas Willis, in 1674 tasted the urine of a patient with diabetes and, finding it to be sweet, reported it as a new characteristic of the condition. More on the redoubtable Englishman later.

One explanation for this may be that information during this period was lost from public view because of the ancient practice and custom of burying precious documents.

Another reason maybe the practice in the ancient civilisations of India and China of hiding precious materials such as these writings in crypts in caves or burying them. Other explanations include their loss over the centuries through destruction by the elements or through deficiencies in the practices employed for their preservation. They may also have been carried off with other spoils by invading armies.

The ancient custom of burying valuable documents was supported by a comparatively recent event which was headlined around the world in the first half of the 20th century and cast an unexpected light on one ancient document in particular, but also on the subject of the preservation of early documents in general. This was the discovery of the Dead Sea Scrolls.

The Dead Sea Scrolls.

In 1947, a Bedouin discovered the first seven Dead Sea scrolls in a cave on the northwestern shores of the Dead Sea. To say that this caused excitement throughout the world particularly in the religious and academic circles of scholars of ancient documents and authorities on anthropology would be an understatement. The writings in these documents were found to be dated back to the time of Jesus either in the century before or the century after his death.

Between early 1950s and 1956 there was keen competition between archaeologists and Bedouins to find more scrolls. The contest culminated in a clear victory for the desert dwellers but the real victors were the scrolls as the final number of manuscripts discovered was in excess of 800.

The material used in the manuscripts included linen and wood but mostly parchment. Since the findings included the period of the pharaohs, the Dead Sea Scrolls also included some manuscripts on papyrus.

In India, the oldest surviving manuscript were written in Sanskrit on palm leaves. These date back to the ninth century, although documents have been discovered, as mentioned later by Barnett in the Joslin textbook (12th edition), which date back to the fifth century.

The discovery of the Dead Sea Scrolls in caves in what was then Palestine and eventually covered a 10-year period between 1946 and 1956, was possibly the result of such practices of protection.

In the Dead Sea Scrolls the contents were Jewish and Hebrew religious manuscripts but similar practices existed to preserve knowledge in other countries as revealed in the Egyptian papyrus.

The mystery of the existence of early documents during this period deepens further when we read of the exploits of the Chinese Buddhist monk Xuanzang in his desert journeys in *The Immeasurable World* (Faber and Faber, 2018) by William Atkins.

Born in 602, Xuanzang had become a novice at 12 years of age, and was recognised by the older members of the Order as being blessed with an exceptional intellect. Following a disagreement with his elders in matters relating to their beliefs in Buddhism, the young man, at the age of 27, travelled to the cradle of Buddhism, namely India. This involved crossing the deserts of China which itself was a journey dreaded by all who knew of it. Undeterred by the many dangers of which he was warned by older members of the religious order, the young monk made his way "guided only by piles of bones and horse dung".

Xuanzang spent 14 years travelling and studying in India, Nepal and Sri Lanka before re-crossing the Taklamakan in the year 645 with twenty-two horses carrying more than 700 works of Buddhist scripture. The contents of such an acquisition are not described in any detail. It is tempting to speculate on the possibility of documents other than religious scriptures being included in such a large quantity of material.

It is possible that more was known, even discovered, about diabetes in the centuries between the time of Aretaeus in the second century A.D. and the English contribution in the 1700s.

As described above, diabetes had been included in the ancient writings of Chinese, Indian, and Korean scholars but the amount of detail in these ancient sources is difficult to come by for various reasons described above. However it is generally believed that the sweet taste of the urine of affected individuals had been described by Indian and Chinese scholars. The reference to diabetes in the Hindu literature dates the documents attributed to Susruta's *Samhita* at around 400 BC. These described the urine as containing honey.

Given the efforts expended on secrecy in the older civilisations in order to preserve and protect valued information it's little wonder that with the end of these periods of history, information on medical and other branches of knowledge was lost not only to their own people of later generations but also to the people of other countries and cultures.

It is thought-provoking nevertheless that in spite of the description of the condition hundreds of years earlier, the details of the main features of diabetes received less emphasis in many of the textbooks of Internal Medicine which are used in the medical schools of English-speaking countries today. This included William Osler's description of diabetes in the textbook of medicine *The Principles and Practice of Medicine* which was published in 1892.

Part Two

European Journeys
After the Long Eclipse

7

THE PERSPICACITY OF ENGLISH PHYSICIANS

The development of and advances in the printing press in the 18th century made a significant contribution to literature in general and medical advances in particular. Technology permitted the making of high quality prints of preserved manuscripts making them accessible to libraries, students and scholars.

An Oxford Professor's Most Unusual Prescription.

Thomas Willis 1621–1675.

Willis, was a contemporary and admirer of Thomas Sydenham (1624–1689), the author of *Observationes Medicae*, which became a standard textbook of medicine for two centuries and led to Sydenham becoming known as "The English Hippocrates."

Willis was possibly unaware of the knowledge of diabetes in the East as contained in untranslated descriptions by Indian and Chinese scholars several centuries earlier which had included descriptions of sweet or "honey" urine.

In 1674 when, in addition to his own practice, Willis was a physician and Professor of Natural Philosophy at Oxford University, he demonstrated what might be considered the ultimate test of a physician engaged in bedside teaching of medical students. To convince, and possibly impress, his students Willis actually tasted a patient's urine. Finding it sweet (and clearly unaware of the Eastern literature mentioned above), he added the word *mellitus* to the already known condition of diabetes. For this reason, diabetes was considered to be due to an abnormality in the kidneys.

In addition to his duties at Oxford University and the teaching of medical students, Willis was also known for his strict instructions to patients who consulted him for their ailments.

It is said that if he discovered a patient had not followed his advice, the professor was not above ordering him out of his office and, for good measure, raining several blows with his walking stick on the non-compliant individual !

Matthew Dobson (1732–1784).

100 years after the observations on the presence of sugar in the urine of a person with diabetes, Matthew Dobson in 1775 boiled the urine of a patient and demonstrated crystals which were brown in colour and tasted sweet. Dobson called this "brown sugar". In 1776 he published his work in *Experiments and Observations on the Urine in Diabetes*.

Dobson's findings reinforced the prevailing view that the organs which harboured the cause of the problem were the kidneys.

The focus on the kidneys as the organ believed to be the "seat" of the condition was to change following the studies of another English scholar.

An Englishman Opposed to British Slave Trade.

John Rollo.

An English Colonial Administrator's Contributions to Diabetes.

> *"I dissuaded him from renting his house and selling his furniture; and, in the most guarded, though effectual manner, told him, that his disease would prove a tedious one, and as it's nature was not well understood, he might be inclined to return and obtain other opinions; and as Woolwich was so near London, the seat of the first medical intelligence, he would prefer, returning. Should the disease not be removed I promised to assist him in every way..."*

An Account of Two Cases of Diabetes by John Rollo.

Rollo, earlier in his career had been in the West Indies in Colonial Administration. A major source of income from that particular British colony was derived from the sugar industry which had employed slave labour from Africa and later, indentured workers from India. Rollo was never comfortable with the slave trade. Later, he had held the position of the Surgeon-General of the Royal Artillery.

Rollo was also a scholar interested in diabetes. He was intrigued by the possibility of sugar playing a role in causing diabetes.

Being aware of the work of Matthew Dobson, he used Dobson's method for measuring urinary glucose and carried out one of the first quantitative metabolic studies in diabetes.

He measured the glucose in his patient's blood and showed that the level was higher than normal thus demonstrating two important features of diabetes: firstly, the presence of sugar in the urine and secondly, a higher than normal level of glucose in the blood (hyperglycaemia).

Using one of his patients, a Captain Meredith whom he described as "a corpulent man with adult onset diabetes and severe bladder coryza," Rollo carried out daily recordings of body weight and the amount and kinds of food eaten, followed by weighing the sugar cake obtained by boiling and evaporating the urine.

These studies showed that different foods changed the amount of sugar lost in the urine.

Rollo wrote a book on diabetes based on his experiments.

> *"An account of two cases of diabetes mellitus with remarks as they arose during the progress of the cure. To which are added a general view of the nature of the disease and it's appropriate treatment."*

The book was published in 1797 and republished some years later.

The importance of Rollo's work was that he changed the thinking on the organ responsible for diabetes and shifted the attention of scholars from the kidneys to the stomach as the "seat" of diabetes.

Rollo suggested that the loss of sugar in the urine reflected an overproduction of sugar from vegetable matter in the stomach and therefore the "morbid" organ of diabetes was not the kidney but the "stomach."

However, the next story reveals a different, important, and previously unrecognised, source of diabetes and challenged the view held at the time that the condition was caused by an unspecified abnormality in the stomach.

Thomas Cawley An Unrecognised "First."

Almost exactly 100 years before Minkowski, and von Mering had demonstrated the role of the pancreas as the "seat"of diabetes in 1889, an English physician called Thomas Cawley in 1788 had reported in detail the post-mortem findings in a patient who had a shrivelled pancreas which contained stones. The patient was known to suffer from diabetes. The authors in the 13th edition of the Joslin textbook commented that this may have been the first published reference to the pancreas in relation to human diabetes, but emphasised that no deductions were drawn as to its possible role as a cause of diabetes.

Frederick William Pavy (1829–1911).

Pavy also described the damage to the nerves especially in the lower limbs of patients who suffered from diabetes.

It is said that Pavy, who worked at London's Guys Hospital, devoted his mornings to consultations on patients with various medical conditions including diabetes, and each afternoon to research. In the evenings he reviewed the results of the day's findings and planned further experiments for his research.

Although complications of diabetes including gangrene and pain from damage to the nerves in feet and legs had been described in early Arabian literature by Avicenna, little progress had been made in clarifying the nature of such conditions. Neither were there any effective measures to alleviate the suffering in those troubled by these complaints in ancient times.

Unfortunately, effective measures for alleviating pain from nerve damage in those suffering from diabetes remains a challenge to this day.

In short, the knowledge of diabetes and especially insulin was at best, incomplete.

Where in the body did insulin come from ?

What was the actual effect of insulin in the body?

Questions such as these continued to trouble not only physicians interested in the condition but the patients and their relatives as well.

Diet was the only treatment and even here there was disagreement over which ingredients were the best.

Harold Percival Himsworth (1905–1993).
Another Forgotten Hero in the Diabetes Story.

The drama of the discovery of insulin, with stories of remarkable rescues, and accounts of the transformation of previously haggard children into healthy, even robust looking individuals was understandably splashed on the front pages of newspapers and magazines throughout the world. No longer was diabetes a death sentence.

Inspite of the clear statement by Frederick Banting and physicians who had been treating patients with diabetes that insulin relieved symptoms but did not cure diabetes, it took some time before the uncomfortable truth was faced.

With the increased lifespan of patients on insulin the effect of diabetes on organs such as the kidneys, the eyes, the heart and lower limbs became increasingly apparent and posed new challenges for the sufferers as well as physicians and researchers.

Important aspect of diabetes especially as it affects middle-aged individuals, owes much to the person who first described it. His name was Harry Himsworth.

Himsworth came from a working class family in Yorkshire, England. His schooling came to an abrupt end at the age of 16, when against their son's will, his parents took him out of school to work in a worsted mill. Himsworth had a sickly disposition. The young man, though compliant, made it clear to his parents that he wanted to continue his education. Somewhat reluctantly they agreed to Harry enrolling in a corresponding course which enabled him to enter University College Hospital in London in 1924 where he started his medical studies.

That Himsworth pursued a highly distinguished career in medical research and later in medical administration is part of the history of the development of medical teaching and research in Britain.

Himsworth's contribution to diabetes has perhaps received less attention than it deserves probably because of his humble and self-deprecating nature.

The essence of his contributions to diabetes, as described in his own words, are found in two lectures he delivered by invitation; the first in 1939, and the second, ten years later.

The 39th Goulstonian Lecture by Himsworth.

Theodore Goulston (1572–1632) was an English physician and scholar. Educated in Oxford University, he was admitted as a Fellow of the College of Physicians in 1611, and was a Censor (examiner) for the College for several years.

In his will Goulston had left £200 which at that time (1632) was a considerable sum, to endow annual lectures which were to be given in the Royal College of Physicians by one of the four youngest Fellows of the College.

In 1939, at the age of 33, Himsworth gave three lectures on the "mechanism of diabetes mellitus."

In 1935, based on his own experiments, Himsworth had provided a definition of Type 1 and Type 2 diabetes which is perhaps more helpful in understanding the difference between the two types of diabetes then the current widely used Type 1 and Type 2 diabetes.

"On the whole the sensitive diabetics tend to be younger and thin, and to have normal blood pressure and normal arteries, and as a rule their disease is of sudden and severe onset. The insensitive diabetics, on the other hand, tend to be elderly and obese, and to have hypertension and arteriosclerosis, and in these patients the onset of the disease is insidious."

10 Years later, in 1949, in the Oliver- Sharpey lecture Himsworth commented on two aspect of diabetes which have become major challenges of the condition not only for those who suffer from this condition, but also for the authorities charged with caring for the large numbers of patients with Type 2 diabetes in the modern era.

In addition to the physiological mechanisms, genetic and environmental factors, which are now recognised as having important roles in causing diabetes, Himsworth also added a cluster of other characteristics including obesity, high blood pressure, high levels of fats (triglycerides) and hardening of the arteries (atherosclerosis). This combination of signs when present in middle-aged and older men and women with diabetes is now referred to as the "metabolic syndrome".

The practical benefit of recognising this is that it alerts the doctor and the patient to the need for taking measures to try to limit, if not prevent, as many of these abnormalities as possible in order to avoid later problems with heart and kidney disease and narrowing or blockage of arteries.

Even in the 1950s Himsworth's views on Type 2 diabetes received little attention.

This was in spite of his observations being confirmed following the discovery of radioimmunoassay namely that in Type 2 diabetes, instead of producing less insulin when given sugar, the patients often produced more insulin. Furthermore, there was minimal emphasis on this in the management of patients with the disorder.

Eventually, when it was accepted that there was a higher level of insulin in patients with Type 2 diabetes to compensate for their comparative insensitivity to insulin, the term *insulin resistance* became an integral part of the definition of diabetes.

Another of Himsworth's observations which now occupies a critical position in the planning of the treatment of Type 2 diabetes was that patients with Type 2 diabetes also have several other conditions. In addition to the higher levels of "blood fats" namelycholesterol and triglycerides. These patients also suffered from "middle obesity" which refers to accumulation of fat around the waist.

This collection of potentially hazardous elements in Type 2 diabetes made such individuals vulnerable to other conditions such as high blood pressure, strokes, heart attacks and kidney failure.

Himsworth's research and findings made all those years ago, are the realities of today's challenges in the management of an increasing number of middle-aged and older patients with Type 2 diabetes.

Thus it may be said that although the discovery of insulin by Banting in 1921 deservedly received worldwide attention, Himsworth's contributions which were made only a few years later, were not recognised for their importance at the time of their discovery.

In fact, Himsworth received due recognition for recognising Type 1 and Type 2 diabetes forty-one years after he had recorded his findings in scientific literature.

Unlike diabetes in children and younger individuals, the condition to which Himsworth made such important contributions, is often treated without the use of insulin.

The modern classification of Type 1 and 2 diabetes arose in 1951 from the observations of physicians headed by John Lister at the Royal Free Hospital which was a women's hospital in Britain. They described a group of women according to their physical characteristics.

The irrepressible Edwin Gale could not resist the tongue-in-cheek comment on the method which may have been used by the researchers to persuade "the tough women" to be measured, weighed - and photographed nude, all in the name of science!

They identified one group of women who had a distinctly different build from the other – a young, thin group with normal blood pressure and a second group with high blood pressure who were older and obese. These they called Type One and Type Two diabetes respectively.

As described above, the distinction had been noted and documented more than a decade earlier by Himsworth.

8

FRENCH SCHOLARS ON JOURNEYS OF DIABETES

"They seek him here they seek him there,
The Frenchies seek him everywhere.
Is he in heaven? Is he in hell?
The damned elusive Pimpernel."

Michel-Eugene Chevreul (1786–1889).

A significant advance in understanding diabetes occurred in 1815 when a French chemist called Michel-Eugene Chevreul (1786–1889) identified the sugar in the urine of a diabetic was glucose.

Claude Bernard (1813 -1878).

"He is not merely a physiologist, he is physiology."

In mid 19th century, two of the most significant events in the history of diabetes were firstly, an opinion expressed by the highly respected French physiologist Claude Bernard (1813–1878) and secondly, a discovery considered central to the story of insulin and diabetes.

Bernard was only too aware of the different opinions held especially by other French scientists on the origin of sugar in the blood. Bernard, who was working in the fabled hospital Hotel Dieu was mentored by François Magendie (1783–1855). Magendie who occupies a permanent place in the history of medicine through the naming of an opening in the base of the human skull named after him as the foramen of Magendie, had written a textbook of physiology in which he stated that "it was impossible to say what is the role of the liquid of the pancreas."

Claude Bernard himself had not been able to successfully remove the pancreas in his own experiments on dogs. He expressed the view that the operation was impossible except by sacrificing the animal.

Bernard therefore changed his focus on experiments on glucose to the way glucose was handled in the liver.

According to some authorities this opinion expressed by the highly respected Bernard may have diverted some research workers from researching the origin of insulin, thus delaying it's discovery.

Gustave Edouard Laguesse (1861–1927).

In 1893, more than 20 years after Langerhans' description of the islets in the pancreas, the French physician and histologist Gustave Edouard Laguesse named these cells, the "islets of Langerhans"

Laguesse, who was born in Dijon (which in modern times is also known for its production of mustard) holds a place in medical history for his contributions to the histology of the pancreas. He's credited with coining the term *endocrinology*, the study of hormones. His research was an important step on the path which eventually lead to the discovery of a new hormone, insulin.

The Frenchman is also accredited with coining the word *endocrinology* to describe the study of the branch of physiology in the human body, which operates through the activity of hormones.

The term *hormone* had been introduced by an English scientist called Starling in 1902, as the name of chemicals in the body which are discharged directly into the bloodstream. The word hormone is derived from Greek meaning "I arouse" or "I stimulate".

In 1910 the Belgian physiologist Jean de Meyer suggested that the product of pancreas which prevented diabetes when isolated from the organ should be called "insulin" which is derived from the "insulae" or islets (of Langerhans).

Insulin continued to frustrate the scientists who were searching for its location. Claude Bernard, one of the most respected French researchers, was aware of the location of insulin in the pancreas because of the work of the German team of Oscar Minkowski and von Mering. However, the exact location of the hormone within the pancreas continued to defy the scientists until it's much publicised discovery by Banting in the small remnant of tissue which was left after the bulk of the pancreas had been destroyed by the digestive juices. If, as was part of the experiment, the duct is tied off, the digestive juice is discharged into the substance of the pancreas and because of its very high acidity, destroys the cells. Since the islets of Langerhans do not share the pancreatic duct or its branches (because they discharge their product directly into the bloodstream), they escape the destruction.

Largely because the islets occupy a very small part of the pancreas, the tiny amount of tissue left after the pancreatic tissue was destroyed was considered unimportant - a critical mistake.

Apollinaire Bouchardat (1806–1886).
In 1883 Bouchardat published a 397- page textbook of diabetes (*De la glycosurie ou diabete sucre*). The French physician, who also worked at Hotel Dieu was generally regarded as a leading authority on diabetes in France. He had observed the effect of weight loss in patients with the diabetes when studying the condition in soldiers who had returned from the Franco–Prussian war of 1870–71. He confirmed this by demonstrating that weight reduction improved diabetes in the obese and therefore emphasised physical exercise as part of the management of the condition.

Bouchardat was among the first to suggest that the pancreas was the primary organ responsible for diabetes. The critical experiment which proved this was carried out in the laboratory of Bernhard Naunyn by Oskar Minkowski (1858–1931) and Josef von Mering (1849 -1908). This is described after the French contributions.

Etienne Lancereaux (1829–1910).
Lancereaux is often forgotten for his contribution to the early literature on diabetes. Based on autopsy and clinical observation he had classified diabetes as *diabete maigre* meaning thin or emaciated

diabetes and *diabete gras,* fat diabetes. More recent examination of his papers have revealed that his patients with "thin diabetes" were emaciated adults with with little resemblance to the juvenile diabetes as understood today. Lancereaux's description of the fat patient with diabetes is consistent with Type Two diabetes of today.

Lancereaux had decided to study medicine because at the age of 20 he had suffered a head injury in a farming accident and was impressed with the medical care he had received. He had mostly studied in Paris.

His reputation was established by a two-volume treatise on syphilis published in 1868–1869 which was immediately translated into English. He continued his remarkable output with the three volume tome Traite d'anatomie pathologique in 1875.

Although a candidate for a professorship, he lost out to Jean-Martin Charcot (1825–1893), the charismatic and highly influential teacher and physician still revered in medical circles throughout the world.

(In the Paris hospital, Salpetriere where Charcot was the Head and Professor of Medicine, the Charcot library preserves his handwritten medical contributions in several hefty tomes.)

Lancereaux's connection in this account is through one of his pupils, Nicolae Paulescu (1869–1931) who had developed an extract of insulin before Banting and Best but was unable to proceed further because of World War I. Paulescu, after completing his medical studies in Paris had served as Lancereaux's intern and assistant before returning to Bucharest.

Lancereaux continued to practise medicine until his death in 1910, following a fall during a visit to a patient's home. He is remembered by the naming of a street in the 8th arrondissement of Paris, Rue du Docteur Lancereaux.

9

TWO MEDICAL STUDENTS, THE REMEMBERED AND THE FORGOTTEN

Two young men, both brilliant medical students and sons of prominent doctors made significant contributions to the early history of diabetes. One is remembered, the other through one of those incomprehensible quirks of history, is seldom mentioned, even in textbooks on diabetes.

Paul Langerhans (1847–1888).
Paul Langerhans came from a respected medical family. His father Paul Augustus Langerhans was a prominent physician in Berlin.

After graduating from high school Langerhans went to the university in Jena, an ancient city described in documents dating back to the ninth century.

Langerhans later transferred to the University of Berlin, and came under the influence and tutorship of the eminent teacher and scientist Rudolph Virchow (1821–1902). Virchow emphasised the value of using the microscope in the study of different parts of the human body. The mantra he emphasised to his students was to "think microscopically."

With hindsight, one cannot help admiring the foresight of the German polymath. He had been quick to recognise the importance of a comparatively new invention, the microscope to gain further insight into the appearance of pathologic material.

On February 18, 1869 Paul Langerhans presented his thesis for a Doctorate in Surgery and Medicine at the Friedrich-Wilhelms University in Berlin.

While studying the cells in the pancreas with the use of the microscope, he had realised that in addition to the well known cells in the pancreas which produce trypsin, a digestive juice, there also existed small clusters of cells which had a different appearance because of their many- sided (polygonal) shape. They looked distinctly different from the rest of the cells in the pancreas. The diligent medical student described the clusters of cells as giving the impression of floating on the surface of the gland.

Langerhans made no further comment on the possibility of the cells providing a secretion or their possible role in diabetes. Neither, for that matter, is there any record of Virchow suggesting any relationship between Langerhans' finding to diabetes.

At the time of this observation, Langerhans was 22 years old.

In 1870, Langerhans served in the Franco-Prussian war. On his return he held the professorship of pathology in Freiburg but shortly afterwards was discovered to have tuberculosis of the kidneys. After an initial response to treatment the young professor failed to regain his health and died in 1888 at the age of 41.

A few years after his death, the islets he described were named after him, guaranteeing him immortality in medical history.

A Medical Student Forgotten by History.

Eugene Lindsay Opie (1873–1971).

The name Paul Langerhans is forever a part of the history of diabetes because of his description of the nest of cells embedded in the pancreas as described above. The name Eugene Lindsay Opie is seldom mentioned. Yet Opie's observation deserves recognition. Like Langerhans', it was also made when Opie was a medical student and had been studying the microscopic anatomy of the pancreas.

Eugene Lindsay Opie (1873–1971) who was in the first graduating class from the John's Hopkins School of Medicine in 1897, added to the observation made by Paul Langerhans in 1869. Langerhans had noticed the difference between the cells in the islets and the rest of the cells which made up most of the pancreas.

Opie went a step further than Langerhans.

Neither Langerhans nor his supervisor, the illustrious Rudolph Virchow had commented on the possible relationship of the islets to diabetes.

Opie made the observation that the islets in patients with diabetes looked different from those in non-diabetic patients.

This provided the link with Minkowski's and von Mering's experiments carried out in 1889 which showed that removal of the pancreas resulted in diabetes. They had failed to recognise that the actual parts of the pancreas responsible were the islets of Langerhans.

When Banting embarked on his project to isolate insulin in 1921, he was clearly aware of the Islets of Langerhans being the source of the hormone.

Opie was born in 1873 in Staunton, Virginia in a medical family. His father Thomas, an obstetrician-gynaecologist, had been one of the founders and deans of the University of Maryland College of Medicine in Baltimore.

Eugene Opie was in the first graduating class of the Johns Hopkins School of Medicine in 1897.

Guided by the highly respected pathologist, William H. Welch, the young medical graduate showed a special aptitude for studying tissue pathology.

As a medical student, Opie had noticed "consistent morphological alterations in the pancreatic islets of Langerhans in patients with diabetes mellitus."

Although these observations were recorded in the *Bulletin of the Johns Hopkins Hospital* in 1900, the body of the article on Opie in Wikipedia stated that the observations had been made when he was a medical student.

As mentioned above, Opie's observations on the changes in the islets of Langerhans in patients with diabetes provided the critical link between Langerhans' observation and the role of the islets in patients with diabetes. This was the missing link after the work of Minkowski and von Mering and the actual relationship of diabetes to a possible abnormality in the islets of Langerhans, something which had been missed by the German scientists who had dismissed as insignificant the small remnant which remained after the destruction of the bulk of the pancreas caused by tying off the gland's main duct.

Two more points of similarity in relation to Opie's contributions to diabetes are that like Frederick Banting and many other young men of that age, he had served in World War 1. He was a colonel in the medical corps and had worked on the prevention of infectious diseases, including influenza and tuberculosis.

Secondly, after leaving Johns Hopkins, Opie moved to New York City and worked in the Rockefeller Institute on subjects not directly related to diabetes. However, his name can be added to the list which contains many other clinicians and researchers prominent in the story of diabetes and insulin who were supported by this institution. These include Frederick Allen who treated diabetes through a carbohydrate restricted diet before the discovery of insulin and Israel Kleiner who isolated insulin before the Toronto group but through circumstances beyond his control, including World War I, was not able to bring his product to the level where it could be used in treating patients with diabetes. This is described later in this account on the controversies following the award of the Nobel Prize to Banting.

(If you can't wait to get to this section, then you have to find the chapter with the title *Whataboutery* p.125).

10

A LANDMARK STUDY
IN GERMANY

"It is a riddle wrapped in a mystery inside an enigma, but perhaps there is a key."

Winston Churchill.

Although Churchill, the cigar-smoking, pugnacious British Prime Minister during World War II, was speaking about Russia, the same could be said about diabetes, a mysterious illness which had been shrouded from scrutiny since the time of the pharaohs of Egypt.

And, at the risk of stretching the analogy, could the key to the riddle inside the mystery be insulin?

The critical experiment which proved that the pancreas was the primary organ responsible for diabetes was carried out in the laboratory of Bernhard Naunyn by Oskar Minkowski (1858 -1931) and Josef von Mering (1849 -1908).

Naunyn is prominent in the history of diabetes, for several reasons as described in a short essay on the eminent professor and mentor in this book.

The experiment which proved critical in the search for the organ responsible for diabetes was the complete removal of the pancreas by Minkowski, who was known for his surgical dexterity. The opinion of the respected Claude Bernard that a total pancreatectomy in a laboratory animal – usually a dog – would invariably lead to the death of the animal had largely put a hold on all attempts to remove the pancreas.

The difficulty in removing the pancreas lies in the gland's blood supply which employs a vast network of very fine, almost thread-like arteries. The surgeon has to exercise great care and caution so as to avoid cutting any of these arteries, which would result in sudden and often uncontrollable bleeding which, as had been Bernard's experience, always led to the death of the animal.

Fortunately for science, Minkowski was not aware of this opinion. Furthermore, the young research scientist was blessed with exceptional manual dexterity.

The operation which was carried out by Minkowski with the help of von Mering's was more than a triumph of surgery.

Contrary to Bernard's pronouncement, the dog survived and thrived – with one problem!

It started urinating frequently. Minkowski castigated the laboratory attendant for not keeping the floor clean only to be told by the young man that the frequency of the passage of urine by "the dog without the pancreas" was so pronounced that he was unable to keep up with the cleaning. Minkowski's curiosity or instinct, perhaps more than scientific perspicacity, led him to test the urine for glucose.

The rest, as the cliché goes, is history.

What is less publicised is that Minkowski and von Mering had carried out two more experiments which confirmed that the pancreas was indeed the 'seat' of diabetes.

Firstly, they grafted a small part of the pancreas which they had removed, back onto the animal which had been passing urine frequently and found that there was an immediate improvement and the frequent passing of urine stopped.

They then removed the piece of grafted pancreas from the same dog and diabetes reappeared.

As recorded in *Joslin's Diabetes Mellitus* (13th edition), the results of their experiments were published in 1889 in the journal Zentralb Klin Med 1889;10:393-394.

An interesting historical fact of this publication lies in the priority ascribed to von Mering presumably by his younger associate, Oskar Minkowski.

As mentioned above, Minkowski was not aware of Claude Bernard's previous studies on the removal of the pancreas in the experimental animal following which the much-respected scientist had failed to keep the dogs alive.

When Minkowski had broached the subject of removing the organ, von Mering told him of Claude Bernard's opinion to which the young man, with confidence verging on bravado, had responded with,"give me a dog."

Von Mering had then obliged with not one, but two animals and assisted his younger associate to perform the operation.

The operation by the experienced and older von Mering coupled with the manual dexterity of Minkowski achieved the successful result which had eluded Claude Bernard.

Many years later, Minkowski admitted that he was unaware of Bernard's opinion on the difficulties of the surgical removal of the pancreas.

Minkowski extended the work begun with the removal of the pancreas in the dogs to an in-depth study on the subject which is now considered a classic. Many consider Minkowski's experiments as the critical steps in the studies which marked the beginning of the end of the early years of the struggle of physicians and researchers to understand the hitherto mysterious condition of diabetes which had plagued the human race for centuries.

Von Mering was the senior member of the team of two in the laboratory, which was under the supervision of the legendary Bernhard Naunyn.

Von Mering had encouraged and supported the younger, enthusiastic Minkowski. They were friends and free of any element of competition between them. It was clear that Minkowski respected his older colleague who was listed as the first author in the now famous publication.

Although perhaps overshadowed by Minkowski in the experiment described here von Mering had made a significant contribution in the field of diabetes four years earlier when he had produced experimental diabetes through the use of phloridzin. von Mering had been taught by and worked with Kussmaul and Hoppe-Seyler. A true aristocrat and a brilliant swordsman, von Mering was appointed

Professor of medicine at Halle in 1890. His book on internal medicine published in 1901 went through four editions before von Mering's death in 1908.

Minkowski also had a high regard for Bernhard Naunyn, his professor and mentor. The story of Naunyn as a mentor to many young physicians including Elliott Joslin, the American pioneer diabetes specialist, is well known.

Minkowski wrote the obituary when Naunyn died in 1925.

Appropriately, the obituary was published in the journal, *Archives of Experimental Pathology and Pharmacology* which had been started by Naunyn who had remained it's editor to the end of his life.

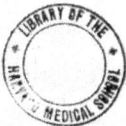

Above is a photograph of the note written by Minkowski to Dr.

Elliott Joslin who had kept in touch with his mentor Naunyn to the end of the latter's life.

The second photograph below is a handwritten letter from Naunyn to Joslin in 1907.

The photograph was obtained from the Harvard medical library by kind permission of the chief librarian Mr J Eckert at the time of my visit to Joslin Clinic and Harvard Medical Library in 2014.

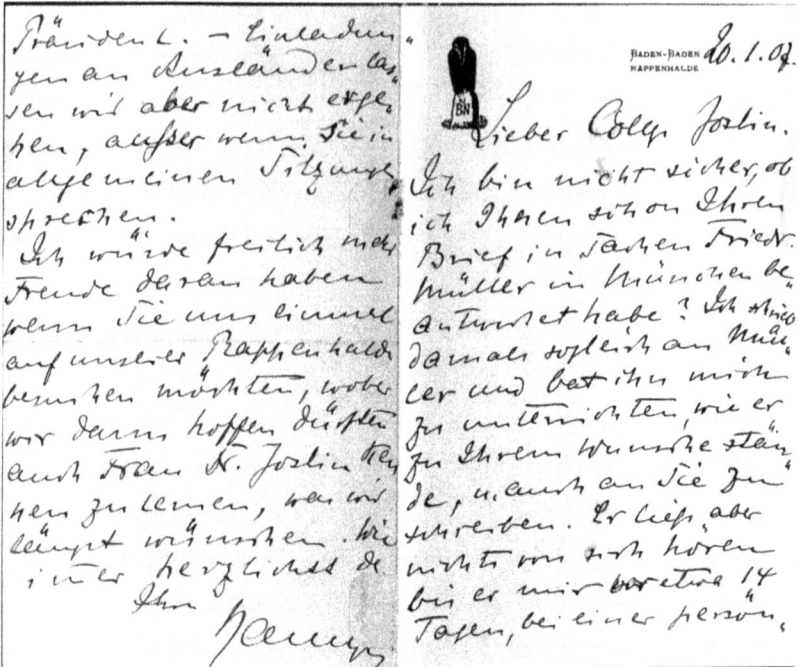

It has been said that Claude Bernard's failure to remove the pancreas was a setback for this area of research until von Mering's and Minkowski's contribution. However, Bernard continued to work in the field and made important observations in the part played by the liver and the brain (pituitary gland) in the way the body handles sugar normally and in a person who develops diabetes.

Bernard used the technique of "*pithing*" which uses a needle to puncture the area being studied. He used a needle to pierce the pituitary gland at the base of the brain.

Students of medical history, especially on the topic of the discovery of insulin, would find it interesting that Frederick Banting had participated in conducting experiments on the pituitary gland under the supervision of the Chief of the Department of Physiology at Western University in Ontario, Canada. Professor F.W. Miller, a respected physiologist and teacher was also the Head of the research department when Banting was working there as a part-time demonstrator in the Department of Surgery.

The findings highlighted by the work of von Mering and Minkowski set the stage for a flurry of activity amongst researchers, especially in Europe and England to find the product of the islets of Langerhans. These researchers believed – and hoped – that this product made in the pancreas could cure the ancient condition which had defied physicians and seers since the time of the pharaohs.

The work galvanised various individuals and teams working on the cause of diabetes.

At this stage, several scientists working in different laboratories, not only in Europe, but also in the United States were pursuing the isolation of the active principle within the pancreas which they hoped would lower blood glucose.

Details of these experiments and the claims which were made, often with some justification, surfaced many years later following the successful isolation of insulin in Toronto.

What happened next took not only the scientific community by surprise, but astounded the entire world.

Part Three

Banting's Triumphant Journey

11

A DAIRY FARMER'S SON. FREDERICK GRANT BANTING

Frederick Grant Banting (1891–1941).

> *"The story of insulin is a story of famous, almost famous and little-known people, of serendipities, discoveries, and re-discoveries. It represents an authentic breakthrough, characterised, at the same time, by contrast, controversies, and disputes, among scholars, as well as by great disappointment, failures, and hopes."*
>
> Ignazio Vecchio et al.

The enigma of diabetes has been aired earlier in this account. Now we will trace the pursuit of the life-changing hormone, insulin.

Until now, dear reader, you have met scientists with impeccable academic pedigrees and accomplishments to match. Now meet a young man who possessed no such distinction. He was not a known researcher. In fact he had virtually no training in medical research. Differences of opinion on the merits of his contribution continue to the present day. Yet history has crowned his contribution and accorded him a peerless prominence at least in the minds of the general public.

After reading this account, you may choose to form your own opinion.

The story begins in the small laboratory of a university in Toronto, a small town of less than half a million people situated in Canada, a

British colony in North America. Toronto had never laid a claim to any particular distinction in scientific endeavour. Yet it is here that we meet a young man who will surprise us in more ways than one.

The story of the discovery of insulin is inextricably linked with one name, Fred Banting.

Frederick Grant Banting was born on November 14, 1891 in Alliston, a small town established in the early 1800s by three brothers, William, John and Dixon Fletcher, who had migrated from England.

The first child born in Alliston was Margaret Grant, the mother of Frederick Banting. She married William Thompson Banting. They had five children and Fred, their youngest, was the only son. The couple ran a dairy farm.

Prior to the discovery of insulin the only medical connection of the Banting family had been through the coincidence of Frederick Banting's father William being baptised by the Reverend Featherstone Lake Osler on the same day as he had performed the same ritual on his own son. By coincidence both boys were given the same first name, William.

William Osler later rose to be Sir William Osler, the famous Canadian physician considered by many to be the father of modern medicine.

The Bantings were a strict Methodist family who attended church regularly, lived thriftily, did not swear, and abstained from smoking tobacco and drinking any form of alcohol. Their social activities were restricted to regular attendance at church and Sunday School. Fred was an awkward dancer and preferred to spend his spare time playing sport, especially athletics. However he was good looking and drawn to Edith, the beautiful daughter of the minister of his church, who became his girlfriend and later, his fiancée. As will be seen later, the engagement and friendship which lasted for many years played an unexpected role in Banting's contribution to the discovery of insulin.

At school Fred was an average student but a good athlete. He kept fit through boxing and running.

Banting's Medical Training.

After completing his high school, Banting went to Toronto University and in 1910 enrolled in an Arts course with the aim of entering the ministry. However, within a year he realised that he was not interested in that branch of studies and switched to Medicine in the autumn of 1912.

Toronto University at that time was a premier medical institution in Canada. The university also housed an impressive research department. However there is no record of Banting engaging in any research apart from what was part of the curriculum (in physiology) during his medical course at Toronto University.

Given his role in the discovery of insulin, it is pertinent to observe that Banting embarked on the quest for insulin with no research pedigree.

Banting's War Service.

World War I (1914 - 1918) played a significant role in Banting's medical training, and indeed in his life. Canada, a British colony, responded to the call to arms. Posters of Lord Kitchener, one of Britain's heroes, exhorted the youth of all the colonies to join the war effort.

The University shortened the medical course from the usual five-year program to 4 years in order to send the young men to enlist in the Canadian army.

Banting was awarded a Bachelor of Medicine degree on December 9, 1916. He reported for duty the following day, December 10, 1916.

After completing his "very deficient medical training" he was sent to serve in the Armed Forces in 1915. Before leaving he became engaged to his girlfriend, Edith Roach.

After a period of training, Banting left for Britain in March the following year. For the first 12 months he remained in Britain at the Grenville Canadian Special Hospital and worked in its Orthopaedics Service.

In June 1918, Banting was transferred to Number 3 Canadian General Hospital in France from where, in August, he was transferred to the 44th Battalion, 4th Canadian Division in Arras. Banting's war service was distinguished.

The battle of Cambrai which was an engagement between the British and German armies is remembered for the carnage caused on both the attacking British and the counter-attacking German armies as well as the large number of lives lost, 12,000 being the official number of casualties recorded by the British and Commonwealth forces. The battle is also remembered for the first full scale use of tanks in warfare.

During this engagement Banting, although wounded, had continued to return fire, refusing to withdraw even when commanded to do so. It is said that amputation of the injured arm was considered but Banting had refused, taking over the management of the wound himself.

He was discharged from the army on December 4, 1918.

In February 1919, Banting was awarded the Military Cross "for courage under fire" in the battle of Cambrai.

The decorated war hero, while convalescing in London, studied and gained a *Membership* (as opposed to a *Fellowship*) of the Royal College of Physicians and Surgeons.

When he returned to Toronto, the restrained Methodist youth of the pre-war years was much more a man of the world, having acquired the worldly vices of heavy smoking, drinking and swearing.

12

THE START OF BANTING'S JOURNEY

Upon his return to Canada in early 1919 Banting was posted to Christie Street Military Hospital. Later, in the same year, he worked with Clarence Starr, the much admired Chief Surgeon at the Hospital for Sick Children in Toronto. Banting was the resident in surgery and became interested in orthopaedics. During his time with Starr, Fred Banting developed a strong and lasting relationship with his supervisor.

After one year of further training as a resident medical officer in paediatric orthopaedic surgery, unfortunately the aspiring surgeon was unable to secure a continuing appointment at the Children's Hospital and, on the advice of Starr, left Toronto and returned to London, Ontario where he planned to work as a general practitioner. He purchased a modest dwelling with funds borrowed from his father. One reason for choosing London was that his fiancé Edith Roach was teaching in a local high school.

On July 1, 1920 the physically imposing, 6 foot tall, 29 year old Frederick Banting, a decorated veteran of World War I, opened his practice in London, Ontario.

At the time London was a small town and Banting had few patients. Often he had days when there were no patients.

According to Michael Bliss's *The Discovery of Insulin* (1982), Banting's total income for July 1920, the first month of his general practice in London, was the princely sum of four dollars.

In addition to the debt he owed to the university for his medical course, Banting had borrowed money from his father to buy the house in which he practised in London. (The house has been preserved as a historic house.)

He tried to save money by not going to the cinema and started cooking his meals at home on the bunsen burner in his dispensary. He built a garage which is where, to while away his idle hours, he began to use oil paints which were to lead to his lifelong interest in painting.

Out of desperation he applied for a part-time position as a demonstrator in surgery at Western University in London. He started there in October 1920. In the new employment Banting was paid two dollars an hour.

Banting's teaching duties at Western University included giving lectures to medical students. Each week started with Banting's lecture on monday morning. Little did he know that this chore was going to prove a turning point in his life.

Banting had become engaged to his long-term girlfriend, Edith Roach, just before reporting for military duties in March 1917. Upon his return, however, the veteran was devastated to discover that Edith's ardour for him had cooled, possibly because Banting himself had also changed from the young man brought up with Methodist traditions to a battle-hardened and decorated veteran. Moreover, his sister Essie had her own reservations about Edith's suitability as Banting's wife.

In mid-October 1920, Edith Roach broke off her engagement to Fred.

Banting, heartbroken, confused and angry, started drinking even more than had been his habit.

Apart from his duties as a demonstrator for medical students, there are few details on Banting's time at Western University with Professor F.O. Miller who was a recognised authority on aspects of human physiology.

The background to Banting's employment at Western University also provides further interesting information on his experience – or lack of it – in medical research. Although much smaller than the Faculty of Medicine in Toronto, Western boasted some good professors. One of these men who was to play a critical role in Banting's academic development and therefore indirectly in the discovery of Insulin was Dr F. O. Miller, who was a very capable Professor of Physiology, and more importantly, a remarkable teacher.

Working with Miller gave Banting, an insight into laboratory research, and Miller's guidance opened the younger man's eyes to the possibilities and rewards for the hours spent in the laboratory.

Arguably, Banting's research may be said to start here because of three incidents.

Miller's method was to stimulate students to engage in animal experiments in order to gain an insight into human physiology.

Secondly, it was with Miller that Banting, as co-author, published his first and only scientific paper in a medical journal before starting on his research on insulin.

Brain: Volume 45, issue 1, June 1, 1922. Observations on Cerebellar Stimulations, by F. O. Miller, MA, MB, and F. G. Banting MC, MB."

Thirdly, it was Miller, who had pointed Banting in the right direction when recently appointed demonstrator, heard expressed an interest in experiments to find insulin. Miller had suggested that Banting seek the guidance of a recognised authority on carbohydrate metabolism namely, Professor James Macleod, Professor of Physiology and Dean of the faculty of Medicine at Toronto University.

It is difficult to escape the conclusion that Frederick Banting embarked on his pursuit of insulin with little, if any experience in laboratory research, one scientist referring to him as having "no research pedigree."

(There is no record of Banting returning to any studies on the pituitary in the years following the discovery of insulin.)

13

A YOUNG MAN'S VISION

"Your old men will have dreams, and your young men will see visions..."

Joel, a biblical prophet and writer.

Banting's duties as a demonstrator at the University involved tutoring medical students. It was during this period that the idea of pursuing the discovery of insulin had occurred to him.

Leaving aside the possibly romanticised stories of the idea occurring in a dream to the rejected suitor Banting – he had recently been told by his long-term fiancé, Edith Roach that she was breaking off their engagement – it was after reading an article in a medical journal in November 1920, that Banting decided on a surgical plan to attempt the isolation of the part within the pancreas which might contain the elusive substance which had been named "insuline" by the English physiologist, Sir Edward Albert Sharpey – Schafer (1850–1935), more than a decade earlier in 1909.

The article which started Banting thinking about isolating insulin was in the November issue of the journal *Surgery Gynaecology and Obstetrics*. The author was a pathologist called Moses Barron, whose work at Mount Sinai Hospital in New York included carrying out post-mortem examinations.

While carrying out an autopsy, Barron had come across a stone which had completely blocked the pancreatic duct. This duct which runs in the middle of the pancreas carries the strongly acidic pancreatic juice out of the gland to the intestine where it is used to digest food.

In his patient Barron noticed that the obstruction of the duct had caused complete destruction of the pancreatic substance but remarkably, the cells of the Islets, which had been described many years earlier by the German medical student Paul Langerhans, had been left intact.

After reading Barron's article Banting had several drinks before retiring. As he was falling asleep, the thought occurred to him that the cells in the islets might contain insulin. He decided to test the hypothesis by tying off the pancreatic ducts – often there's more than one duct in the pancreas – in experimental animals (dogs) to see if he could isolate the Islets of Langerhans and extract insulin from them to treat diabetes in human beings.

He wrote down the basic steps in the surgical approach needed to carry out the procedure. The piece of paper on which the sketchy experimental plan was written down by Banting has been preserved in the archives of Toronto University and is quoted later in this account.

The next morning Banting approached Miller to discuss the project of isolating insulin he had envisioned the previous night. Miller indicated to the aspiring researcher that Western University did not have the required facilities for the experiments proposed by Banting. He pointed out the necessity for large animals for experiments on the pancreas. Dogs had been used most commonly for this purpose, especially by the French physiologist, Eduard Hedon whose work on the effects of removing the pancreas of dogs was well known. Furthermore, Miller was aware of a world authority on diabetes who by fortunate coincidence happened to be in Toronto. James Macleod, Professor of Physiology and Dean of the Faculty of Medicine at the University of Toronto was the obvious man to approach for guidance in what Banting was contemplating.

Banting immediately set to work and secured an appointment with the professor a week after Miller's suggestion.

Neither man could have known that the contemplated partnership, seemingly made in heaven, was going to end in the way it did as immortalised in the history of the discovery of insulin.

John James Rickard Macleod (1876–1935).

There is scant mention in the recorded history of the discovery of insulin of Macleod's impeccable academic credentials or a record of his publications directly related to diabetes and insulin. Unlike Banting, Macleod had been an outstanding student in his undergraduate years. In 1898 he had graduated with honours in the medical course from Marischal College in Aberdeen. He had then pursued studies in Leipzig University, one of the oldest and most prestigious educational institutions in Germany which counts amongst it's alumni, the musicians Robert Schumann and Richard Wagner as well as the poet Goethe and, in recent times, the retired Chancellor of Germany, Angela Merkel.

Macleod had returned in 1900 to lecture on Physiology and Biochemistry at London Hospital Medical School. In 1903 he had been appointed Professor of Physiology at Western Reserve University, (now called Case Western Reserve University) in Cleveland, Ohio. It was here that he did most of his research on the pathology of diabetes.

His publications on the subject established the reputation of the medical school. In 1913 Macleod had published a monograph, *Diabetes: It's Pathological Physiology.* This was followed in 1918 by *Physiology and Biochemistry in Modern Medicine.*

In 1918, he was invited to the Professorship of Physiology at the University of Toronto.

Macleod returned to Scotland in 1928, to accept the prestigious Regius Professorship of Physiology at his alma mater Marischal College where he stayed until his retirement.

Macleod had married Mary Watson McWalter in July 1903. They did not have any children.

James Macleod died in 1935 and was buried in Aberdeen.

Possibly due to the adverse publicity associated with him sharing the Nobel Prize with Banting, Macleod had few honours bestowed on him in Canada. Belatedly in 2021, he was inducted in Canada's Walk of Fame.

Macleod's Assistance to Banting in the Quest for Insulin.

Whether or not Banting realised that he had "struck gold" in discovering an expert on the very subject he was pursuing has not been discussed in any of the writings on the subject of insulin. Suffice it to say that within a few days of hearing from Banting, Macleod had written him a letter dated March 11,1921 inviting him to discuss the matter with him in person on May 15, 1921. In that letter Macleod explained that because of Easter holidays and University examinations it would be best for Banting to start on May 15.

There are no details on any discussion relating to previous research on diabetes during that initial meeting between Macleod and Banting. Had Miller told Banting about Macleod's publications? Did Macleod ask Banting about his knowledge of previous research on diabetes? In his reply to Banting and Best when told of the promising results they had achieved following the injection of the extract in dog number 408, Macleod had mentioned the work of Israel Kleiner. Given that Bliss had spoken of Banting "having read widely on the subject of carbohydrate metabolism, and even read a little about diabetes," had there been any discussion between Macleod and Banting during that initial meeting on Banting's knowledge of the subject which he wanted to investigate?

Many such questions of obvious importance in the account on the discovery of insulin, and specifically on the relationship between Banting and Macleod have been obscured by the emphasis on the disagreements between the two men. Little had been written about this aspect of the insulin story until the book by Michael Bliss. As a historian, Bliss concentrated on what he considered would be of interest to the general reader. Charles Best had been a student in the science course taught by Macleod. Did Best tell Banting about Macleod's academic distinctions and experience including his writings on diabetes? One of the textbooks used in the course, which Best had just completed had been written by Macleod. Surprisingly, even current literature in medical journals or historical accounts has not addressed these questions. In 1913, Macleod had written a book on diabetes, *Diabetes: It's Pathological Physiology* which was published in

London by the prestigious firm of Longmans Green, & Co. This part of the insulin story is uniform in its lack of this aspect of Macleod's experience and knowledge of diabetes and insulin as existed at the time when Banting embarked on his search for the elusive hormone.

At no stage during his studies or hospital duties had Banting shown any interest in biochemistry, medical research or diabetes. His residency in the Children's Hospital had been largely to do with orthopaedics. Indeed in later years Banting commented that he recalled one of his classmates at university having diabetes, but that is where his acquaintance with the condition seemed to start and end. Certainly he had never treated any patient afflicted with the condition.

In his memoir, *The Story of Insulin* published in 1940, Banting recorded his recollections of that night.

"I was disturbed and could not sleep. I thought about the lecture and about the article, and I thought about my miseries and how I would like to get out of debt and away from worry. Finally about two in the morning after the lecture and the article had been chasing each other through my mind for some time, the idea occurred to me that the experimental ligation of the duct and subsequent degradation of a portion of the pancreas, one might obtain the internal secretion free from the external secretion. I got up and wrote down the idea and spent most of the night thinking about it."

The account in the memoir is more expansive compared to the notes in Banting's notebook housed in the Academy of Medicine in Toronto, and quoted in *The Discovery of Insulin* by Michael Bliss in 1982:

"Diabetus" (*sic*).

"Ligate pancreatic duct of dog. Keep dogs alive until acini degenerate leaving islets.

Try to isolate the internal secretion of these to relieve glycosuria."

Perhaps more by chance than through reasoning based on research or academic studies of carbohydrate metabolism in general or diabetes in particular, Banting had concluded that the internal secretion might relieve glycosuria (the loss of sugar in the urine).

In drawing this conclusion Banting was ahead of the more experienced Moses Barron who, in a letter to the young researcher two years later in February 1923 said, "Although I was quite interested in the study of the pancreas at the time when I published that article, I did not have the faintest idea or hope that it would be at any time or in any way be sufficiently suggestive to start such an epoch-making investigation as you have undertaken. Barron went on to say, "I feel it an honour to be in anyway mentioned in connection with this work of yours, and I wish that I had actually had some real part in the investigation."

Banting's Plan of Action, or Lack of It.

Banting had little, if any training in medical research. Neither is there any evidence of him being interested in that branch of learning. Remember that his position at Western University had been sought and obtained simply as a way to supplement his income from medical practice.

That he was working in the department headed by F.O. Miller has had a hitherto largely unappreciated role in the insulin story. Miller, a highly respected physiologist was also active in research when Banting had approached him with his idea. Miller quickly identified two important issues which Banting needed to address. Firstly, he told Banting that the experiments he was contemplating would require larger animals than were available at Western. Being unfamiliar with previous work done on the search for insulin, especially by European workers including the French physiologist Eduard Hedon, Banting was unaware that most of the research had been carried out on dogs.

Secondly, Miller suggested to the aspiring researcher that the work he was contemplating would require the guidance of one who was experienced in the field of carbohydrate metabolism. Being familiar with the literature on the subject Miller told Banting that a man highly respected in that field happened to the head of the Department of Physiology at the very medical school from where Banting had graduated, namely Toronto University.

That man was John James Ricard Macleod. Prior to his appointment in Toronto, Macleod had been the Professor of Physiology at Western Reserve University in Cleveland, Ohio, USA.

He had been interested in the metabolism of starches in the human body in general and diabetes in particular as far back as 1905. He was also familiar with the research carried out by earlier workers, including Minkowski. Macleod himself had carried out experiments to investigate the role of the brain causing the blood sugar levels to rise. He knew that the pancreas was the "seat" of diabetes but, like many other workers in the field, had not been able to demonstrate just what the pancreas actually did, or did not do, to cause diabetes in an individual.

Thus the contact suggested by Miller to Banting to explore the aspiring researcher's idea would appear, at least on paper, to be a godsend. Unfortunately as the story unfolds, it will be seen that the association between Macleod and Banting turned out to be anything but cordial.

Within a week of receiving Miller's advice, Banting had set up an appointment to see Professor Macleod in Toronto.

Details of that meeting held on November 7, 1920 have escaped the scrutiny of the majority, if not all those who have written on the subject. There is no record of Macleod ascertaining Banting's knowledge of the part played by carbohydrates in nutrition and other aspects of human physiology. Neither is there any record of Banting being aware of Macleod's academic accomplishments nor that fact the learned professor had actually written a book on diabetes.

At the end of the meeting, Macleod agreed to let Banting use the facilities in the Department of Physiology laboratory during the summer, when most of the members of the staff, including Macleod were going to be on holidays.

Banting, beside himself with anticipation, returned to London, Ontario to dispose of most of his possessions within days, then packed his essential belongings into his car and relocated to Toronto.

The next meeting with Macleod was held in April 1921 when he was provided with laboratory space, two dogs, and a student helper who had completed a course in physiology, (but had not at the time submitted his thesis).

The student was Charles Herbert Best.

Given his experience in experimental work, Macleod must have harboured some doubts about Banting succeeding in his quest. However to his credit, Macleod gave the aspiring researcher an opportunity to pursue his idea.

As the Dean of the faculty of medicine, Macleod was conscious of his responsibility towards the university, and was concerned about the use of dogs in experiments being carried out by Banting, an inexperienced researcher.

The use of animals for experiments at the time was being vigorously opposed by sections of the community generally known as the anti-vivisectionist movement. One incident which was prominent in the public eye was known as the Brown Dog Affair.

The Brown Dog Affair.

> *"If this is not torture, let Mr Bayliss and his friends...tell us in Heaven's name, what torture is."*
>
> Stephen Coleridge.

The reason for including this in some detail is that several well known medical men as well as prominent literary figures feature in the story. In addition, more than one individual in the Brown Dog Affair also had a role in the insulin story.

Ernest Starling (1866–1927) features prominently in medical textbooks. The Professor of Physiology at University College London and his brother-in-law, William Bayliss. (1860–1924) were said to be "compulsive experimenters" who used vivisection in Starling's laboratory. Starling is well known for his medical contributions, including coining the term *hormone* from the Greek root meaning "I arouse" or "I excite." (Insulin is a hormone).

The operation on the brown dog, which was central to the Brown Dog Affair also featured a medical student who carried the dog out of the lecture theatre when Bayliss had finished. The medical student was Henry Dale, later Sir Henry Dale who had been dispatched to Toronto charged with the responsibility of checking on the merits or otherwise of the discovery of insulin.

Prominent literary figures of the time who also feature in the story through their support or otherwise of the antivivisection movement included the writers Thomas Hardy and Rudyard Kipling. The story was carried by the radical newspaper *Daily News* which had been founded in 1846 by Charles Dickens.

Mark Twain, an antivivisectionist, published a short story, *A Dog's Tail* in Harper's magazine in December, 1903.

In 1903, Sir William Bayliss, a professor of physiology at University College, London, performed an operation (vivisection) on a brown terrier-dog before an audience of about sixty medical students. Although the animal had been anaesthetised, two Swedish women who were members of the Anti-Vivisection Movement and had managed to get into the lecture hall to witness the demonstration, claimed that the anaesthetic was inadequate.

The antivivisection movement in the period 1860 to 1910 was a group mostly led by women, many of whom were also prominent in the fight for women's rights. The movement was opposed to use of animals for scientific purposes. It had widespread support among animal lovers, including Queen Victoria, the British monarch at the time.

The incident involving Bayliss became a political controversy, which raged in Britain between 1903 and 1910 and led to two Royal Commissions.

Stephen Coleridge, a descendant of the famous poet Samuel Taylor Coleridge, was vehemently opposed to animal experiments and publicly accused William Bayliss for having broken the law during the experiment. Bayliss sued for libel and was awarded £2000 in damages.

Antivivisectionists commissioned a bronze statue of the brown dog as a memorial which was unveiled on the recreation ground in Battersea in 1906. The plaque on the statue read, "Men and women of England, how long shall these things be?"

The medical students considered this provocative and promptly tore down the statue and the plaque.

The Brown Dog affair became a political controversy on vivisection and remained prominent in public discussion between 1903 and 1910. it was still very much in the public consciousness during the time of the research on insulin.

14

BANTING'S SURGICAL EXPERIMENTS

Details of various aspects of the pursuit of insulin by Banting have been described in the book *The Discovery Of Insulin* (University of Chicago Press) written by the late Michael Bliss and released in 1982.

Bliss, a historian said,

> *"I want to reconstruct the discovery of insulin research dog my dog, day by day, experiment by experiment."*
>
> (Italics by the writer).

Bliss, a historian with no knowledge of, or experience in, science or medical research had to rely on interviews with physicians and researchers for the medical aspects of his book.

Leaving aside the many colourful aspects of the happenings in the laboratory such as Banting's tirades against anyone he suspected of interfering with his project, he and Best spent much of the summer of 1921 in pursuit of insulin.

The search for insulin started on May 17, 1921 when Banting operated on the first dog. Macleod assisted in what was a difficult operation perhaps as much to support the young researcher (considering that Banting's experience in surgery was largely in orthopaedics) as to satisfy himself that adequate care was being taken. Macleod had impressed on Banting the risks of surgery on account of the very rich and profuse blood supply of the pancreas.

Unless the larger arteries were avoided and the smaller ones tied off, the possibility of severe haemorrhage and the death of the animal was a constant danger.

There is no record of Macleod taking part in any surgery after this. A month later, in mid June 1921, the professor left for his usual annual summer holidays in Scotland. He returned to Toronto three months later and resumed work on September 21, 1921.

It is important, however, to record the essential contribution of Macleod as well as several others whose help and support enabled Banting to start and complete the project.

This is acknowledged in an early paper written by Banting and Best in the *Journal of Laboratory and Clinical Medicine* in February 1922.

"The hypothesis underlying this series of experiments was first formulated by one of us in November 1920, while reading an article dealing with the relation of the Isles (*sic*) of Langerhans to diabetes. From the passage in the article which gives a resume of degenerative changes in the acini of the pancreas following ligation of the duct, the idea presented itself that since the acini, but not the islet tissue, degenerate after this operation, advantage might be taken of this fact to prepare an active extract of islet tissue. The subsidiary hypothesis was that trypsinogen or its derivatives were antagonistic to the internal secretion of the gland. The failures of other investigators in this much- worked field were thus accounted for.

The feasibility of the hypothesis having been recognised by Professor G. J. R. Macleod, work was begun under his direction in February 1921, in the Physiological Laboratory of the University of Toronto. Help was also generously rendered by Professors Henderson, Fitzgerald, Graham, and Defries."

The experimental work which showed that an extract made from animal pancreas reduced the loss of sugar in the urine of the experimental animals had been carried out while Macleod was away in Scotland on holidays and maybe summarised as follows:

Banting followed the operating methods firstly of Hedon whose method involved removing the animal pancreas through a two-stage procedure. Later, he used the one-stage operation described by Francis Madison Allen in his *Glycosuria and Diabetes,* an 1179-page tome with more than 1200 references which had been published in 1913 by Harvard University Press. At the time Allen was one of the most influential American specialists on diabetes.

After several failures, most of them from infection causing the death of the dogs after operation, on July 30, 1921 Banting and Best found that the pancreatic extract they had prepared and injected into dog number 410 had lowered the glucose level in the animal's blood.

In early August both researchers wrote to Macleod, who was still on holidays to report their success.

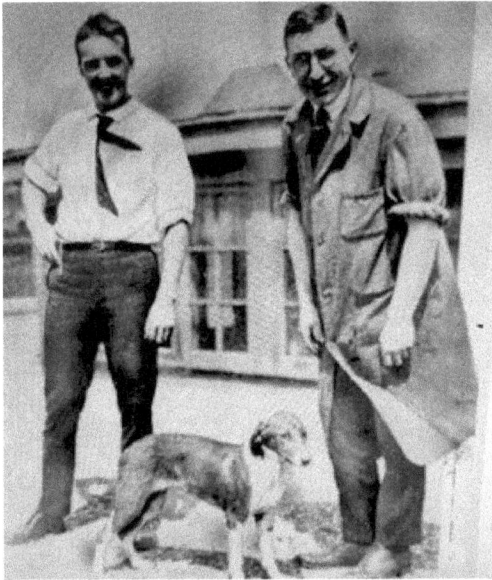

Banting (on the right) and Best with the dog
successfully treated with the pancreatic extract.

Macleod replied and cautioned against premature celebrations. He urged them to repeat their experiments. Also, for the first time, he referred to the work of Israel Kleiner who had isolated an effective pancreatic extract. Kleiner's work is described later in this account.

On August 15, 1921, two dogs – number 92 number 409 after having had their pancreases removed were treated differently. 92 was given the extract and dog 409 was not. The following morning the dog which had been treated was thriving. The untreated dog had died.

Banting was convinced that he had found insulin. Macleod was still on holidays. The researchers did not do any further work and waited for the professor to return.

15

THE FIRST PRESENTATION OF THE DISCOVERY OF INSULIN

Upon his return, Macleod looked at Banting's work and suggested that he present his findings at the University's Journal club. This was an informal meeting of an in-house group of researchers and clinicians who worked in different parts of the University and hospital as well as the research laboratories which were part of the campus. Although small, the group often included senior physicians, surgeons, and researchers who, though involved in projects of their own, wanted to hear of work being done by others in the various University/ Hospital departments.

The first presentation of the results of the experiments to the Journal Club was, as Banting had hoped, on his 30th birthday.

Banting described the procedures and the results. Best showed the slides.

The presentation produced two important results.

Firstly, Norman Burke Taylor (1885–1972), an experienced physiologist asked if a long-term (longevity) experiment had been considered.

It had not.

Given that the treatment of diabetes was indeed long-term, this was an important aspect of the project which needed to be addressed.

Banting and Best embarked on it within 48 hours.

The second outcome which also had far-reaching consequences was through two individuals who were there for their own very different reasons.

The first was JHA Clowes, a high-ranking employee of the pharmaceutical company Lilly. Clowse was in charge of the production of pharmaceuticals as well as their marketing. The appeal of insulin for the treatment of diabetes would have been obvious. Clowes, who was always on the lookout for products with a potential for marketing, recognised it immediately in the Toronto researchers' discovery.

In the area of commercial pharmacy, no one in Toronto University's Department of Physiology, including the professor, was in the same league as the Lilly operative.

We will meet him more than once in the insulin story.

The second individual at the Journal club meeting was Llewellis Franklin Barker who at that time was on the staff of the Johns Hopkins Hospital. Barker was in the habit of visiting his alma mater whenever he returned to Toronto. He recognised the potential of the findings of the two young researchers and related the finding to anyone he met.

The word spread quickly.

Marjorie the Dog of Special Fame.

The longevity experiment on dog 33, later given the name Marjorie, was begun on December 6, 1921. The first animal, dog 27 in the longevity experiment had died, possibly from anaphylactic shock.

Marjorie not only survived, but thrived for 70 days while receiving daily injections of the extract. In spite of the criticisms expressed, the longevity experiment was generally regarded as having been successful.

The effective extract was made through the expertise of James Bertram Collip, a visiting professor from the Rockefeller Foundation. Collip had joined Banting and Best before Christmas 1921, after they had isolated the extract which had lowered the blood glucose level in experimental dogs. Collip, an accomplished biochemist, was in Toronto on a three–month Rockefeller Travelling Fellowship to work with Macleod in the Department of Physiology at Toronto University.

After a few false starts, the extract was injected in a 14-year-old boy called Leonard Thompson on January 22, 1922. It produced a remarkable response. The blood sugar fell to normal levels and, perhaps more importantly, the patient "felt better."

Before the discovery of insulin Thompson had survived on the Allen starvation diet for some seven or eight years, but was feeble and markedly underweight. It is unlikely that he'd have survived much longer had it not been for insulin.

After starting on insulin he had worked in a drug and chemical company.

Thompson died in a coma after an emergency admission to the Toronto General Hospital in1935.

Daily injections of Insulin had given him a comparatively normal life for thirteen years.

By February 1922 the extract was being tested on patients in Toronto General Hospital.

16

AN EPOCH-MAKING ANNOUNCEMENT

The Summer of 1921. The Dawn of a New Era.

> *"Now there is no longer a need to say "hope long deferred maketh the heart sick" because of the young Lochinvars of Toronto. All praise to them and to Canadian medicine. The practical ingenuity of the New World has here distanced the Old World hypotheses on intermediary metabolism...*
>
> *Pisgah's heights have been ascended and the Promised Land is in plain view."*
>
> *Elliott P Joslin. The Shattuck Lecture, 1922.*

The Association of American Physicians had been established in 1885 by seven physicians, but mainly driven in its formation by William Osler and William Henry Welch, professors of medicine and pathology respectively, who were at that time working at the Johns Hopkins Hospital in Baltimore, Maryland.

The stated aim for its establishment was "to inspire the full breadth of physician-led research across all fields of science related to medicine and health for improving patient care and the health of Americans."

On May 3rd, 1922, at a meeting of the Association of American physicians, James Macleod presented a paper with the title "The Effect Produced on Diabetes by Extracts of Pancreas." The authors listed were Frederick Banting, Charles Best, Bertram Collip, Walter Campbell, A. Fletcher, James Macleod and E. C. Noble. A transcript of the discussion in which various members of the audience had participated was published.

The most important paper on the subject had been published in February of that year in the *Journal of Laboratory and Clinical Medicine, VII,5 (February 1922): 256–271*. The title of the paper was "The Internal Secretion of the Pancreas." The authors were Banting, Frederick G. and Best, C. H.

Thus the results of the work begun by Banting with his assistant Charles Best on May17, 1921 were announced to the medical world by James Macleod on May 3, 1922.

To say that the response to the presentation was enthusiastic would be an understatement. The audience, made up for the most part, of conservative senior physicians and professors gave a standing ovation at the end of the presentation by Macleod, a first in the history of that staid organisation.

Solomon Solis-Cohen (1857–1948), a professor at Jefferson medical College at the time, was effusive in his comment saying, "this study, so careful and comprehensive, this work, so thorough in its execution, and so clear in his presentation, may justly be called epoch-making. I am glad that I have been privileged to hear that paper."

Francis Madison Allen was typically generous, but also precise and, intentionally or otherwise, precise in his praise saying, "If, as seems to be the case, the Toronto workers have the internal secretion of the pancreas, fairly free from the toxic material, they hold unquestionable priority for one of the greatest achievement of modern medicine, and no one has a right to divide the credit with them."

Given his background in research into the nature of diabetes including his comprehensive study contained in Glycosuria and Diabetes, an 1179 page tome with more than 1200 references published in 1913, Allen may well have been aware of the attempts of other workers, including those in Europe, to isolate an effective pancreatic extract. If he was hoping to head off challenges based on the priority rules of scientific publishing, history would show that little attention was paid to his remarks.

Rollin Woodyatt, who had been active in diabetes research in his laboratories in Chicago, declared that he was convinced of the value of Banting and Best's findings. He said that the Toronto group had been able to extract the internal secretion of the pancreas.

"I think that this work marks the beginning of a new phase in the study and treatment of diabetes. It would be difficult to overestimate the ultimate significance of such a step."

Even Woodyatt, admired for his intellectual prowess, could not have dreamt of how prophetic his pronouncement was to prove.

Even 50 years later, Walter Campbell, one of the physicians from Toronto General Hospital where the early trials had taken place said, "we had made it." Campbell had been present at the meeting.

Regardless of varying opinions on the methods used by Banting, and the credit given to him, there is general agreement on the discovery of insulin being a landmark in medical history.

It saved, and continues to save the lives of millions around the world. It restored to health countless men, women, and children who were emaciated to an extent difficult to imagine in today's world.

Larger scale production of the extract for use in patients was obtained largely through the cooperation of the Lilly Company.

Dramatic stories of the changes brought about by insulin injections in patients who were often within days or weeks of dying emerged from Canada, United States and later, from other countries.

Accolades and honours were lavishly bestowed on the discoverers, especially Banting and Best.

Canada basked in the glory.

Banting was knighted.

Then, as if all this weren't enough, the 1923 Nobel Prize for Physiology or Medicine was awarded to Frederick Banting, at that time the youngest to receive the honour. It was shared with James Macleod.

Controversies over the sharing, and indeed the award to Banting, continue to this day with many dissenting views.

One of the more balanced opinions to answer some of the criticisms of Banting's and Best's work on insulin came from an unlikely, and non-medical, source.

In 2003 Henry Bruce Macleod Best, the younger son of Charles Best wrote a book with the title *Margaret and Charlie. The Personal Story of Dr. Charles Best, the Co-Discoverer of Insulin.*

The 500-page work largely drawn from the voluminous archives kept by Charles Best and his wife Margaret Mahon Best covered a period which began when Best was a student and before their marriage in 1924 and ended after both he and his wife had died– Charles in 1978 at the age of 79 and Margaret in 1988, aged 88. Both of them had been avid letter writers. Margaret Best who had been in the same class as Charles in high school (and had always beaten her classmate in the annual examinations) was an excellent diarist and record keeper.

Henry Best, the second of their two sons, was a retired historian. He had also been the President of Laurentian University and had spent some time in Canadian national politics as the Executive Assistant to the Secretary of State for External Affairs. At the time of his writing *Margaret and Charlie,* Henry Best was 66 years old.

Henry Best addressed several criticisms levelled at the work on insulin done at the time of its discovery in Toronto.

The first was his comment on the first "public" presentation of the results of Banting's and Best's research at the American Physiological Society's conference held at Yale University in New Haven, Connecticut on the afternoon of Friday, December 30, 1921. To say that this had not gone well, especially from Banting's point of view, would be an understatement. Inexperienced at public speaking, he himself admitted that he had not done well. His halting presentation had to be rescued by Macleod, who was an experienced and accomplished speaker who had been presenting papers at scientific conferences for many years.

It was at this conference when Macleod, in all probability unintentionally, when answering questions from the audience offended Banting by referring to the work presented having been done by the Toronto team. Banting claimed that Macleod had unfairly taken a share of the credit for the work.

To the end of his life he waged a campaign of trenchant criticism of the Head of the Department of Physiology.

Henry Best, using his years of experience at the University, was much more forgiving of the two young researchers as far as the presentation at New Haven went.

He said, "...the importance of the reports lay, not in the form, but the substance".

Elaborating on this later, he said, "in succeeding years, there have been harsh criticisms of the weaknesses in the early papers. Flaws there were, certainly, but the result was of world- shaking importance, and that is what mattered. The lack of experience of Banting and Best, the initially poor working conditions and lack of financial and other support make that achievement all the more impressive."

Henry Best's summary of the insulin story is worth quoting, if for no other reason than it's brevity because it condenses the entire exercise of the discovery of insulin, from the beginning to the end, in one sentence.

"Thus ended an extraordinary two and half years in the University of Toronto, beginning with the pioneering work of Banting and Best in the summer of 1921, followed by the nerve- wracking but exciting period of development, purification, and manufacture of insulin in 1922, to the rollercoaster ride of recognition, controversy, and honours in 1923."

The controversy and honours refer to the Nobel Prize awarded to Banting and Macleod in 1923. This is dealt with in another part of this book.

Given the exhaustive process of implementing the research findings into clinical practice today, one can only view with amazement the entire process which began with the first experiment on 17 May 1921 being completed on May 3rd, 1922.

It had taken barely a year to discover the extract of insulin which was to transform the lives of millions.

In spite of the enthusiastic reception accorded the presentation by respected authorities in the field, criticisms of various aspects of the work carried out in Toronto, expressed at the time have continued to. simmer ever since.

Insulin removed forever the life-sentence which had from the beginning of time hung over the future of the sufferers namely, the inevitability of an early death.

Insulin gave the patients and their families the remarkable gift of hope. No longer did diabetes mean an inexorable downhill course culminating in the loss of the lives of the young people so affected.

Now, after thousands of years in obscurity, insulin had been brought out of the shadows and placed squarely, front and centre, on the world stage.

There are many references to the unmitigated joy which accompanied the relief experienced bye physicians who had treated diabetes before the discovery of insulin. Foremost among these were Elliott Joslin of Boston and Francis Allen of the Rockefeller Hospital in New York.

Joslin, a devout Christian, compared the transformation achieved by the use of insulin to the imaginary transformation in the Valley of Bones in the bible.

A similar biblical reference was made by Sir Derek Dunlop, Professor of Therapeutics and Clinical Medicine in Edinburgh, who declared that he had "… never seen anything in medicine, more heartwarming or rewarding than to watch those diabetic patients raise themselves step by step out of the valley of the shadow…."

Undoubtedly, the discovery of insulin in Toronto was the dawn of a new era in the emerging drama of diabetes.

17

A SECRET UNAUTHORISED TRIAL OF INSULIN

The first trial of insulin on a human patient was a secret known only to the discoverer of insulin, Frederick Banting as related earlier, Banting had graduated in Medicine at the University of Toronto in Canada just before the beginning of the Second World War. In fact the medical course had been shortened in order to get the young graduates off to Europe to serve in the army. To say that he was inexperienced in medical research let alone in trialling a new medication on patients ("clinical trials"), would be an understatement.

Being the only practising doctor in the team of four who were involved in the pursuit of insulin Banting was impatient to use it on a human patient suffering from diabetes. Even though most of the experiments had been carried out on dogs, the young researcher was convinced that insulin which had reduced the level of blood sugar in these animals which had been made diabetic by the surgical removal of their pancreases could well produce a similar effect in humans.

He fully realised the difficulties inherent in getting a human guinea pig – until he remembered one of his classmates in medical school. His name was Joe Gilchrist.

Gilchrist was known to suffer from diabetes which had been diagnosed in 1917, when he was in the Canadian Army Medical Corps. He had been treated with the Allen diet which was the only treatment available for patients with diabetes at that time.

Gilchrist, like Banting and the rest of the class of 1917, had to report for duty immediately after graduation from medical school. Their course had been shortened from the usual six years to five so that they could contribute to the war effort.

Banting lost no time in contacting Gilchrist and phoned him on December 20, 1921. Understandably, the young man was only too willing to be the human guinea pig. Anything which held the promise of relief from the day–to–day challenges of treatment, and the ever–present risk of diabetic coma with the strong possibility of death, was worth trying.

Banting had always first tried the different extracts prepared from experimental animals by injecting himself before giving them to anyone else. This time he decided to give Joe Gilchrist the extract by mouth, possibly to spare his classmate the pain of an injection.

The young doctor swallowed his friend's magic potion on December 21.

According to Michael Bliss's account in *The Discovery of Insulin,* the incident is documented (in Banting's handwriting) on an index card in the Banting Papers preserved in the Archives at the University of Toronto as follows:

> "December 20, phoned Joe Gilchrist. – Gave him extract that we knew to be potent – by mouth – empty stomach. December 21 – no beneficial result."

Just how the enthusiastic researcher decided how much of the extract to give Gilchrist has not been described in his own or any other account from that time. Suffice it to say that the extract had no effect whatsoever on the blood sugar level in Gilchrist. The reason for this is that insulin taken by mouth is destroyed by the strong acids normally present in the stomach to help digestion. Therefore, Banting's magic potion was destroyed before it could be absorbed into the bloodstream.

Medical history records that when a satisfactory preparation of insulin was eventually developed, Joe Gilchrist was one of the first patients to receive it – this time by injection !

Saved by Insulin. The Later Life of Joe Gilchrist.

After his graduation in 1916, Gilchrist worked with Banting in the clinic at Christie Street Hospital. The building had originally been a cash-register factory but was converted so that it could be used as a facility devoted to treating patients with diabetes.

Gilchrist spent the rest of his working life as Banting's assistant. He was often left to treat the entire group of patients because Banting was in constant demand to lecture on the newly discovered treatment and was often away in different parts of Canada and the United States.

It was also left to Gilchrist to lecture to patients and train dieticians and nurses in practical day-to- day exercises such as learning the method to determine blood sugar levels, preparing the needles for injection by sterilising them first, and the actual technique of giving insulin by injection.

The Toronto Star which had 'scooped' the story of the discovery and gained worldwide prominence as a result, remained in touch with the Christie Street Clinic and therefore with Gilchrist, who was frequently quoted in the paper.

Gilchrist continued at the Christie Street clinic for many years after the death of Fred Banting in 1941, but eventually retired.

He never forgot Banting's loyalty and friendship, often recalling that Banting had assured him that he had "a job for life" and had sealed the undertaking by "shaking on it."

Gilchrist jokingly referred to himself as "a human rabbit" in the the discovery of insulin by Banting.

Eventually, worn down by years of long hours at work as well as frequent hypoglycaemic reactions, Gilchrist stopped working.

Given the furore over the credit for the discovery of insulin especially after awarding part of the Nobel Prize to Macleod in 1923, one can only speculate on Gilchrist's feelings. He had been, as stated by Banting himself, "in the very centre of the pursuit of insulin."

Not only had Gilchrist been the human volunteer, or, as he referred to himself, "the human rabbit," but he had also contributed to the knowledge of the practical aspects of the use of the hormone in the earliest period of its trials on patients with diabetes.

Thinking of the end of Gilchrist's time at the Christie Street Clinic, one is reminded of a Cormac McCarthy phrase describing a man with "a vivid past and an uncertain future".

Little is known about Gilchrist's professional life after leaving the Christie Street Clinic. His home life was turbulent especially as he became increasingly dependent on alcohol. Sadly, eventually his marriage had ended in divorce.

In 1951, Gilchrist was admitted to Sunnybrook Hospital in Toronto, this time not as a doctor, but a patient.

By this time, his diabetes and its treatment with insulin injections had taken a heavy toll. The once muscular limbs and full buttocks carried the scarring of the skin and the hollows where insulin injections had been given over the years. The hollows were an early side-effect of insulin injections caused by the shrinking of the tissues under the skin (atrophy) where the insulin injections were given. He had managed to control his diabetes quite well, but at the time of his admission, he had signs of heart failure.

Joe Gilchrist died in 1951 at the age of 58 years. He was often referred to as "the first walking diabetic patient to receive insulin."

Banting who had died before Gilchrist, never forgot his classmate's contribution to the work on insulin. He said, "it was on him that we tried out not only new batches of insulin but many experiments…, the time in relation to meals…and the treatment of overdose of insulin."

18

ABRAHAM LINCOLN'S CALL TO ARMS

Insulin in the Market Place. Enter the Merchant.

Overcoming the obstacles in the laboratory in the course of finding the most effective way to isolate the extract from the pancreases of animals was a major achievement. This had been achieved by many workers as has been described in this story.

However there was much more to be done to the insulin extract before it could be given to the thousands of patients with diabetes not only in Canada and America but throughout the world.

Taking Insulin from the research laboratory to the patient is an oft forgotten aspect of the insulin story.

Therefore it is appropriate at this point, to introduce an important player in the drama. It is here that we meet men who in effect were merchants, but who recognised the importance of the discovery of insulin, not only for its commercial potential but for the wider benefit of the suffering thousands.

Without their help it is doubtful if the Toronto workers would have been able to develop their product to the the required degree of purity and in the quantities required for the large numbers of patients who needed to be treated.

Foremost amongst those whose cooperation led to the delivery of insulin to the masses was a pharmaceutical company. If luck, as many believe it to be an important element of success in business, is to be counted as a factor in Banting's delivery of insulin, then it is the contribution made by a company which began through the efforts of an early chemist, an apothecary. The story is worth telling for more than it's role in the discovery of insulin in Toronto.

The Lilly Company also features prominently in the story of the "modern" insulin described next in this work. The company retains its place as one of the major pharmaceutical concerns in the world today.

The Good Samaritan Drugstore in Indiana.

Eli Lilly, born in 1838, was the eldest of 11 children of Gustavus and his wife, Esther Kirby Lilly who lived in Greencastle, Indiana.

In 1854, the 16 year-old Eli travelled 60 miles by train from Greencastle to visit his uncle Caleb Lilly and aunt Hennie in a town called Lafayette in the state of Indiana.

Eli was fascinated by the many stores in the thriving town. For some reason, one particular shop attracted him. It was called the Good Samaritan Drugstore. He was fascinated by the strange scents and aromas which were entirely unknown to the recently graduated university student. Eli told his uncle Caleb about the store where he said he would like to work. The owner Henry Lawrence was known to his uncle as a man of upright character.

The apothecary agreed to employ Eli as an apprentice. Eli's jobs included sweeping the floors, caring for and clearing the fireplace, washing bottles and jars, stacking shelves, and running messages and other errands. Also included in his list of tasks was to take care of Henry Lawrence's horse. Eli was paid one or two dollars per week, plus "keep."

In the evenings Eli read whatever books were available on the subject of pharmacy. After a year's training he was permitted to mix drugs.

The diligent apprentice left Lawrence after earning a certificate of proficiency. He then worked in different pharmacies, including a wholesale drug business, in different towns in Indianapolis.

In January 1861, with some financial assistance from his parents plus his own savings, Eli Lilly opened a drugstore on the town square of Greencastle. Also, in January 1861, he married his childhood sweetheart, Emily Lemon.

Unfortunately for Eli's business, President Abraham Lincoln called for his supporters to take up arms to join the Civil War in April 1861. Placing civic duty above his love for his young wife and his new business, like many other Americans who had strong convictions on such issues, Lilly answered the call. Locking the door of his drug store, he bade Emily goodbye, and joined the infantry.

After the war, Lilly ran a 1400 acre cotton plantation in the south at Port Gibson Mississippi. African slaves were the chief source of labour, especially in the cotton fields.

The business venture failed and around the same time his wife Emilie died, possibly as a complication of malaria from which Eli and his son Josiah had also suffered.

In 1867, Eli returned to his profession and worked as a chemist in the wholesale drug house of Harrison Daley and Company.

In May 1876, at the age of 38, Eli Lilly opened a business with himself as a sole proprietor. It was probably the smallest pharmaceutical plant in the United States.

From these humble beginnings, the Eli Lilly company has become one of the worlds most prominent manufacturers of pharmaceuticals and veterinary supplies. It's critical role in the Insulin story began even before the discovery of the hormone in 1921.

Unfortunately Eli Lilly died on June 6, 1898 after a year's illness. The Indianapolis news editorial said of him, "He freely gave his means; he gave more freely still of his personal endeavour."

Josiah Kirby Lilly Sr, "J.K" (1861–1948) born in Greencastle, Indiana, was the only son and heir of Eli Lilly.

After his graduation from the school or pharmacy, JK became the superintendent of the Lilly Laboratories in 1882 before assuming the presidency of the company after his father's death in 1898.

From the point of view of the insulin story it is important to note that during his leadership, Eli Lilly's son introduced strict and high standards of manufacturing. The father had told the son of his own commercial failures. JK never forgot the lessons.

Pertinent to the discovery of insulin was the decision taken by Lilly to significantly increase the research efforts of his company to develop new drugs. He employed an Englishman who was a trained scientist and experienced researcher. Furthermore, the new addition to the Lilly Company was no shrinking violet when it came to the profit motive. JHA Clowes was to play a critical role not only during the development of insulin by the Toronto group but also in its manufacturing for commercial distribution by the company to hospitals, physicians and patients.

The Lilly Company's early association with the discoverers of insulin has continued which has given the pharmaceutical company a leading role in the marketing of, and research into the newer forms of the hormone used by patients and prescribed by physicians around the world.

19

INSULIN DELIVERED

A fact not sufficiently emphasised is the generosity of the Toronto team in making insulin freely available throughout the world. Patents were granted and the method of production detailed for individuals, companies and countries.

Stories abound of parents with children suffering from diabetes writing to Banting for help. They were encouraged by the Canadian to continue on the strict diet and were sent supplies of insulin as soon as it had become available. Banting's thoughtfulness and conscientiousness in this regard has not received sufficient emphasis in the literature. Nor was his attention to the needy restricted to patients in Canada or the neighbouring countries including England and the United States.

A recent article in the Medical Journal of Australia by S.Templer recounted the story of a five-year-old girl in Adelaide, South Australia whose father was sent supplies of insulin by Banting in 1922.

Five-year old Phyllis Adams was the first Australian to receive insulin. She had developed diabetes eight months earlier, and was surviving on severely restricted rations. Her father, having heard of the work being done in Toronto, had written to Banting who had urged the concerned parents to persist with the restricted diet because he and his fellow-researchers were at that time testing the pancreatic extract on dogs.

The little girl who grew into adulthood and motherhood gained a place in the Guinness Book of World Records for having survived for 76 years with the help of daily injections of insulin.

Further refinements and improvements in insulin so as to enable patients to use the longer-acting preparations less frequently than every 2 to 4 hours throughout the day became the next goal of the teams of research chemists.

In 1936 a Danish doctor called Hans Christian Hagedorn (1874–1949) developed the first of these. Protamine Zinc Insulin lasted longer than 24 hours.

The relief of the many problems associated with insulin up to that point was such that the Boston physician Elliott Proctor Joslin, a leading authority on diabetes at the time, hailed the introduction of the new preparation as the beginning of a new era in the treatment of diabetes, which he called the Hagedorn Era.

However Protamine Zinc Insulin (PZI) is no longer in use for various reasons, including the unpredictability of its duration in individuals and also because of severe low blood sugar reactions.

Hagedorn later developed medium acting insulins including the popular NPH insulin which carry his name (Neutral Protamine Hagedorn) and remain one of the most popular insulin preparations used throughout the world.

In 1950, the introduction of *sulphonylurea* tablets to lower blood sugar was a major advance in the management of diabetes especially in adults suffering from Type 2 Diabetes. Today the most widely used tablet for the control of diabetes in adults in most countries around the world is *Metformin*.

Recently, much public attention has been drawn to the widespread use of one of the modern medications for the treatment of diabetes in adults.

Newspapers and other news media have publicised Ozempic, a trade name for a recently developed medication which needs to be injected once a week to lower blood glucose levels in patients with diabetes. It is also effective in causing weight loss and has been used for this purpose by some individuals who do not have diabetes.

The publicity has been caused by its use by non-diabetic individuals to lose weight leading in some countries to a shortage in supplies for patients with diabetes.

In addition to improvements in medications for diabetes there have also been marked advances in methods of delivery of insulin which has enabled patients to take it through automated devices, thus freeing them from using injections. Similarly, implanted devices now enable continuous monitoring of the glucose levels. Unfortunately, in the poorer countries the cost of some of the modern methods of insulin delivery are beyond the means of many patients.

20

CANADA'S FIRST NOBEL LAUREATE. THE NAME MOST REMEMBERED

Richer by far is the heart's adoration…
Dearer are the prayers of the poor.

Richard Heber 1811.

In a telegram from Stockholm dated October 25, 1923, carried by the Canadian Pacific Railway Company addressed to Dr. Frederick G. Banting announced that

> *"the Royal Caroline Institute has presented to you together with Professor Macleod The Nobel Prize of the year 1923."*

Frederick Banting and James Macleod were jointly awarded the Nobel prize for Physiology or Medicine. Banting was, and remains, the youngest winner of the award in the division of Physiology or Medicine.

In his Nobel lecture delivered on September 15, 1925 Banting was generous in acknowledging the assistance of many physicians and scientists including those from the United States, who had become aware of the importance of the discovery of insulin from the meeting in New Haven on December 30, 1921.

An even bigger audience had been present at the formal "epoch-making" announcement of the discovery in a paper delivered at the medical conference of the Association of American Physicians held in Washington DC on May 3rd, 1922.

To say that this announcement set alight the medical fraternity of the United States would be an understatement.

The press was quick to publicise the news and reported again the dramatic findings.

The English-speaking world was just as quick to recognise the importance of the discovery made in Toronto.

Doctors, patients, parents, friends and relatives of those afflicted with diabetes wanted immediate supplies of the wonder drug. Some of the dramatic stories during this early period of the discovery are included in this account.

A recurring theme, especially in medical reports was Banting's and Best's work on insulin taking only 12 months to complete. Today's medical researchers would not contemplate such a short period of time to complete the study like the one undertaken by the Toronto team. Just the requirements which have to satisfy the various committees in research centres and hospitals even before starting any research project can take more than 12 months.

Banting's Life in the Limelight. 1921–1941.

The successful treatment of a patient with diabetes as demonstrated in Toronto in January 1922 had been preceded by reports in medical journals followed within weeks by newspapers around the world.

Although the news item was carried by the major newspapers around the world, it's effect on the scientific community is perhaps not as well known to the layman.

Within weeks of the award different sections, at least in the medical community, freely expressed differing opinions as to who should have been given the prize. Opinions on whether Banting or Macleod alone was entitled to the recognition had different "champions."

Toronto, or for that matter the entire country of Canada embarked on celebrating "our Nobel Prize" with gusto.

"Congratulations" the newspapers trumpeted, fanning the outpouring of self-praise. Politicians were quick and vocal as they also gloried in the triumph of the researchers but were quick to attribute the discovery to the effort of the whole country – *our* scientists, a *Canadian breakthrough* etc. etc.

Dinners and banquets became the order of the day with politicians and society matrons who were assigned seats at the head table, jostling for positions next to the discoverers especially the younger "tall, good-looking" Fred Banting.

Local and national honours followed ranging from a stamp featuring Banting, to his photograph appearing on the cover of Time magazine in August 1923. The once financially strapped, part time demonstrator in the the Department of Surgery at Western University, now received a handsomely-salaried lifelong position at the University of Toronto.

21

A SHORT INTERVIEW ON THE SHORES OF SYDNEY HARBOUR

On the 22nd of January last year (2022) which was the centenary of the first injection of insulin in a human patient who had diabetes, I went for a walk on Balmoral beach which is located near Sydney harbour in Australia.

During summer Sydney is a popular destination for tourists escaping from the winter of the northern hemisphere.

On that day there were several groups relaxing on the beach and the surrounding grassy areas.

On an impulse, I walked up to a young man, probably in his late 20s, and asked him if he knew what insulin was.

"*Yes,*" he said.

"Do you know what it's used for," I asked. He shrugged his shoulders, then pointed to his upper arm "*Diabetes* ?"

"Yes," I said."Do you know who discovered Insulin?"

He shook his head, *no*.

"Never mind," I said. "Are you enjoying Sydney?" to which he nodded his assent.

I walked away.

A minute later I heard a voice, "*Bunting (sic)* ?"

He returned my smile when I asked where he was from "Spain".

Admittedly, the insulin in use today is very different from the preparation which came out of the original work of the team in

Toronto in 1921. However there is no argument that regardless of all the refinements and changes it has undergone, the pancreatic hormone was, and still is, at the centre of the treatment of diabetes especially Type One diabetes.

In spite of the claims and counterclaims, the fact remains that Frederick Banting's name is, and always will be, linked with the discovery of insulin.

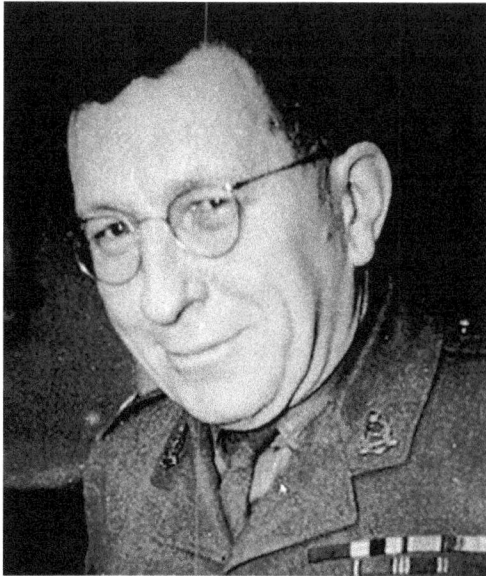

Sir Frederick Banting (1891–1941).

22

"THE PRIORITY RULE."
A LESS SAVOURY ASPECT OF
THE INSULIN STORY

There has been a continuing controversy over whether Banting and his colleagues were the *first* to discover insulin.

This is related to what is often referred to as the "Priority Rule" in scientific publications. Arguments over the individual or a group making a discovery before anyone else have occurred more than once in the scientific literature over the years. A related issue is whether the researcher has *published* his or her findings first.

In today's world with easier access to publishing in most countries due to the advances made in communication and especially since English became the preferred language of scientific literature the question of who has published a certain finding before anyone else is more easily addressed.

The situation was different in earlier times when the exchange of information between scientists and researchers in one country with other workers in the same field in another country was not as easy because scientists and physicians usually wrote in their own language and, as was the case with the team in Toronto, did not speak any other language. They published their findings in scientific journals which used English.

Two Historic Clashes over Claims of Priority.

"I was first" is not a new claim in scientific circles. Here are two examples of such claims made and waged by men who were prominent in the their particular fields of science.

The Calculus Controversy.

Isaac Newton versus Gottfried von Leibniz.

As far back as the 17th Century, there are written accounts of a bitter clash between the Englishman Isaac Newton (1643–1727) and the German polymath Gottfried von Leibniz (1646–1716) on who was the first to develop calculus, a branch of mathematics.

Newton had first published his work on the subject in 1666. They were contained in his book, *Principia Mathematica*, which was published in 1686.

Arguments began with Gottfried von Leibniz, a precocious student and polymath who had taught himself Latin at the age of eight and then, because he was bored, had taught himself Greek. By the age of 14 he had completed his bachelors degree in philosophy and then a masters in the same subject two years later. In 1665 when 17 years old, he was awarded a bachelors degree in law.

Leibniz's interest in mathematics started at the age of 25. Records of his work on calculus in the year 1675 are preserved in the manuscripts in his notebooks.

Leibniz did not publish any of his mathematical works on calculus until 1684, two years before Newton's book was published.

Each man had his supporters whose vociferous accusations of plagiarism were levelled at one of the scientists.

As in the Nobel saga over the discovery of insulin, national pride trumped objective analysis. Although the German had published his work before Newton, the English supporters accused him of plagiarising Newton's unpublished ideas. In Germany the opposite view had overwhelming support.

Eventually the matter reached an uncomfortable resolution largely because Georg Ludwig of Hanover, who had been Leibniz's patron became King George I of Great Britain in 1714. However, Leibniz was still in disfavour - at least in England - at the time of his death in 1716. Sadly, Newton could not rise above his relentless and vicious attacks on Leibniz even after the German prodigy's death.

Later, the consensus moved to a position of the two mathematicians having independently developed and described calculus in Europe in the 17th century.

Charles Darwin's Tantrum.

Darwin (1809–1882) V Gregor Mendel (1822–1884).

Given the importance of heredity and later, the prominence of the gene in this work, questions of priority in earlier experiments and observations on heredity are of interest.

A much publicised disagreement followed Darwin's claim that Mendel had plagiarised his work led to heated arguments between the two giants of science.

Darwin, who unlike Mendel, came from a wealthy English family, was afforded the luxury of travel. In 1831, when he was only 22 years old, Darwin received an invitation to work as a naturalist on the HMS Beagle commanded by Captain Fitzroy. During a trip which lasted nearly 5 years the ship surveyed the coast of South America during which time Darwin explored parts of the continent in the nearby islands, including the Galapagos. He visited many parts of the world, including Australia, between January and March 1836. In Australia the young man travelled over the Blue Mountains, in a north-westerly direction from Sydney to the town of Bathurst. It has been speculated that seeing the mountain ranges, an ancient land, may have played a part in Darwin contradicting the biblical version of God creating the earth.

The reason for the fight with Mendel was Darwin's book, *The Origin of the Species* which was issued on the 22nd November, 1859. (The initial batch of 1250 copies was said to have been snapped up in a matter of days).

Gregor Mendel (1822–1884), a quiet monk who led an ascetic Spartan life, published his observations as *"Experiments in Plant Hybridisation"* in the Proceedings of the Natural Historical Society of Brunn in 1866.

Mendel had presented his findings to the Natural History Society a year earlier on February 8, 1865.

Darwin accused Mendel of copying his work which was vehemently rejected by the monk.

Even though it later became clear that each man had come his conclusions on inheritance independently, the issue was never resolved between the two scientists and only explained by scholars many years after both Darwin and Mendel had died.

A simple explanation for Darwin's quarrel with Mendel is found in the biography of Darwin (*Darwin* by Adrian Desmond and James Moore). It appears the Darwin had somewhat limited linguistic capabilities with no knowledge of any language other than English. This prevented him from reading Mendel's work.

The difficulties encountered by Banting and Best because of their limited knowledge of languages other than English was an important reason for the work of European scientists not being taken into account when they were conducting their own experiments in Toronto.

Returning to the controversy over the discovery of insulin, I have selected the work of one scientist to describe many of the hurdles which had to be overcome in the course of the search for the elusive pancreatic product before the results of the experiments could be published.

After this there is a brief description of the work of other researchers who had also made significant discoveries related to the isolation of insulin before the success achieved by the team in Toronto.

23

WHEN MY IPHONE "PINGED"
LATE AT NIGHT

At 5:30 am on May 8, 1994, a young scientist found a gene which he had been searching for over the previous eight years. He was only 39 years old.

The gene he discovered produces a hormone which plays an important role in obesity. The discoverer of the gene called that hormone *leptin*, which comes from the Greek word for "thin".

Today, if you asked anyone at all familiar with research on obesity, they will tell you that young researcher's name. Jeffrey Friedman.

During my preparation for this work, I had come across an article on the discovery of insulin published in a magazine for general circulation.

When I saw the name of the writer, I recognised it as the name of a scientist I had read about some years earlier but didn't think he was the the author of the piece in the magazine until I saw his comment on his own scientific background. Friedman's facility with words and his lucid explanation of complex scientific information (related to insulin) was impressive.

One fact, which had always stayed with me since I had first read of Dr. Friedman's work now came back.

And it was this, the experience of making a discovery, especially when it has taken years of spending long hours in the laboratory is never forgotten by the individual engaged in the pursuit. Earlier in this story there was unmitigated joy when James "Bert" Collip had isolated insulin in a powdered form during his time with Banting towards the end of December 1921. He said, "I experienced then and there all alone in the top storey of the old Pathology Building perhaps the greatest thrill which has ever been given me to realise."

More commonly the discovery appeals to the eye of the scientist.

John Jacob Abel's spontaneous reaction to the first sighting of insulin crystals coating the inside of a glass jar in his laboratory in December 1925 was a breathless exclamation.

"One of the most beautiful sites of my life," he had said.

A similar experience was described by Herb Boyer in his research related to modern insulin which you will find in the second part of this work.

Friedman's Eureka moment on that Sunday morning which marked the end of a pursuit which had taken eight, yes eight years was

"It was astonishingly beautiful."

It was after 10 at night when I found an email address at the Rockefeller Centre and somewhat hesitantly sent an email to Professor Friedman for permission to use part of the material in his essay. I was not sure if I had the right address or if Dr. Friedman would even respond to what after all was a "cold call." Barely ten minutes after I had sent my email, I heard my iphone *ping.*

Dr. Friedman's permission to use the information from his article was gracious and generous.

I soon realised that his essay was written with such control and discipline that it was going to be difficult, at least for me, to summarise it.

24

A MODERN DAY PROFESSOR'S PERSONAL ODYSSEY

"Discoveries are delicate things."
Jeffrey Friedman, the discoverer of Leptin.

Friedman's article chronicles the work of Israel Kleiner who had discovered insulin at least eight years before Banting. The story explains the circumstances which resulted in Kleiner's failure to carry his work to completion. Some of the factors which caused the young researcher's discovery to be denied the recognition it deserved, also applied to other researchers who were engaged in looking for insulin before Banting.

All these experiments were carried out before Banting's. Remember that Banting was still in medical school when World War I started.

Friedman's lucid exposition of the work of Israel Kleiner demystified the technical details of the search for insulin and made it easier for the reader to understand the experiments carried out by researchers who had pursued insulin with varying degrees of success before the discovery by the Toronto group.

Professor Friedman's interest was piqued by an account of Kleiner's research on insulin in the book *The Discovery of Insulin* written by the historian Michael Bliss and perhaps also because Kleiner had worked at the Rockefeller Institute where Friedman works. The institution is now called the Rockefeller Hospital.

The scientist contacted the author to ask about the Kleiner's later work but found that Bliss could not provide any details beyond the brief description provided in his book. Bliss admitted that he had not followed up on Kleiner's academic life or research after the discovery of insulin.

Bliss's account had mentioned Kleiner's work as part of the contribution made by a number of scientists who had been engaged in the pursuit of the elusive hormone.

Friedman's interest had been further aroused by the paucity of information on the young man. Kleiner would have been in his early 30s at the time of his research at the Institute.

Friedman wrote that he then decided to embark on "a personal odyssey to understand the forces that had both shaped and limited Kleiner."

He hoped that these forces might explain the circumstances which had prevented Kleiner from discovering insulin long before the Toronto team had.

A Brief History of The Rockefeller Institute and its Contribution to Diabetes.

The current Rockefeller University began life in 1901 as The Rockefeller Institute for Medical Research. It was financed and founded by John Davidson Rockefeller (1839–1937), leader of the Standard Oil Company who has been considered by some to be the wealthiest man of all time. He was also known for his philanthropy.

In 1958, the Institute changed its name to The Rockefeller Institute. On the advice of, and in collaboration with, William Welch, a professor at the Johns Hopkins Medical School, who was considered one of the medical giants of the period and later known as "the Dean of American Medicine", Rockefeller established the Rockefeller University and provided the funds needed for research and associated activities including patient care in its hospital.

The Rockefeller University was one of the first American institutions to focus on biomedical investigation. It was before the time when the government allocated funds for such bodies. For the research community, the Institute was a godsend.

Today, more than a century since its beginnings, the institution continues its original "mission" of financing and promoting medical research in many disciplines.

The role of this long-standing institution in the insulin story has not been highlighted in any previous account of the history of diabetes or of insulin.

One of the leading specialists in diabetes in the early years was Frederick Allen who was a physician to patients with diabetes admitted to the hospital attached to the Rockefeller Institute. Allen pioneered the treatment of diabetes with the low–calorie diet often referred to as the "Allen diet" which, for practical purposes, was the only treatment which could be offered to patients with Type One diabetes in the years before the discovery of insulin.

In Banting's quest for insulin, an early association of the Rockefeller influence was through James Bertram Collip who had joined Banting while on a Travelling Fellowship granted by the Rockefeller Foundation. Collip refined the pancreatic extract to a standard which allowed its use in patients with diabetes without causing the problems of infection and unpredictable effectiveness as had happened with the extract prepared by Banting and Best.

An earlier association of this institution was with Eugene Opie (1873–1971) who as a student had documented the difference in appearance between the cells in the Islets of Langerhans. In 1904 Opie had moved from Johns Hopkins to the Rockefeller Institute, but had worked in areas unrelated to diabetes. In addition to working as a pathologist, Opie at that time was also an editor of the *Journal of Experimental Medicine.*

25

ISRAEL KLEINER'S EXPERIMENTS AND WORLD WAR I

...."*while great discoveries are obvious in hindsight, it is considerably more difficult to discern one in the making.*"
Jeffrey Friedman on the discovery of insulin by
Israel Kleiner (1885–1966).

Kleiner, a grandson of Jewish immigrants, had grown up in New Haven, Connecticut and attended Yale as an undergraduate. He was drawn to biochemistry as well as metabolism. Biochemistry was the branch of science pioneered by Russell Chittenden. The highly regarded scientist and teacher had first included that subject in the course of studies at Yale. Chittenden's successor, Lafayette Mendel, a pioneer in the science of nutrition, had supervised Kleiner's studies in researching glucose metabolism.

The young man's star was in the ascendancy when he completed his PhD in 1909 and the following year secured an appointment to the Rockefeller Institute.

Kleiner joined the Rockefeller Institute in 1910 when he was 25 years old. For the young researcher, this proved a golden opportunity. His supervisor was Samuel J.Meltzer, a Russian-born, German-trained physiologist, who was already well known for having invented one of the earliest respirators, a device to help the breathing of patients with lung disease. He was supervising and overseeing a variety of physiological experiments on different organ systems, and agreed with, indeed encouraged Kleiner, to continue the studies on glucose which the young graduate had been engaged in when working with Mendel at Yale.

In the early 1900s, diabetes was not as prominent in public consciousness as it is today except for the one "face" of the condition. This was diabetes in children, the so-called Type One diabetes. Apart from the so-called starvation diet, which itself caused the child to become thin and weak, there was no treatment at that time. The child lost his or her life within 1 to 2 years, often in a matter of months. Stated bluntly, the condition was tantamount to a death sentence.

The pursuit of the exact mechanism which caused the high levels of glucose in the blood in diabetes became the focus of Kleiner's studies.

In 1913 Kleiner and Meltzer, working with dogs made diabetic by the removal of the pancreas, showed that when these animals were injected with glucose the concentration of sugar in the blood reached very high levels compared with the levels obtained in dogs which were not diabetic.

In their next experiment they injected an extract of the pancreas at the same time as injecting glucose in their diabetic dogs.

They found that in the second experiment the blood glucose level did not rise.

Thus, eight years before the discovery of insulin by Banting, Kleiner had clearly demonstrated that the pancreatic extract he had prepared reduced the blood glucose level in experimental diabetic animals.

These findings were reported in a meeting of the National Academy of Sciences in Washington, which attracted a front page headline in the *New York Times*: *Found Diabetes Cause, Now Find a Cure.*

In order to study the methods being used in Europe to investigate this problem, Kleiner left for the continent in June 1914. He was visiting laboratories in Germany, England, and Denmark when a calamity ensued which was soon to engulf much of the western world.

On 28 June 1914, Franz Ferdinand, the heir presumptive to the throne of Austria–Hungary was assassinated in Sarajevo by a 19-year-old Bosnian called Gavrilo Princip. This single act precipitated a series of historic events which within four weeks of the assassination led to World War I starting on 28 July 1914, and ending with an armistice on 11 November 1918.

The huge toll of death and suffering was due to the escalation of military action through the involvement of several other countries.

Figures for the total human cost of this bloody conflict vary, but generally are in the order of nine million soldiers killed and 23 million wounded in combat. Other estimates put the total figure of lives lost and of the wounded close to 40 million.

The war also took a heavy toll on civilians, five million of whom died from consequences of military action and other privations such as disease and starvation.

Kleiner, who was travelling with his family, checked into a quiet hotel in Paris but soon felt "besieged" by the frequent questioning about their nationality by authorities and strangers alike.

"It soon became so dangerous in Paris, that we thought of nothing but getting out," he told a newspaper when he returned to America.

Together with his family, Kleiner had managed to board a New York–bound steamer within hours of World War I being declared.

The effect of World War I on research into diabetes in general and insulin in particular came to the fore in the controversy generated by the 1923 Nobel Prize for Medicine and Physiology which was awarded to two of the four individuals most closely connected with the discovery.

Since the most important part of Kleiner's work on insulin was done at the Rockefeller, the changes made at this centre because of World War I directly affected Kleiner's research.

The Effect of World War I on Research at the Rockefeller.

Rockefeller Institute's first director, Simon Flexner, the brother of the prominent educator Abraham Flexner, was also a friend of Rockefeller. The industrial magnate gave him free reign in making decisions regarding appointments to the Institute.

According to Professor Jeffrey Friedman, Flexner was attracted to scientists with an established reputation. He assembled an international cast of distinguished scientists involved in medical research.

For example, Alexis Carrel, a Frenchman was engaged in developing innovative techniques to improve surgical procedures achievers methods of suturing and procedures, useful in organ transplantation. In 1912 Carrel won the Nobel Prize for Physiology or Medicine. He was the first scientist working in America to receive the Nobel Prize.

Attached to the Institute was the Rockefeller Hospital, which became the first research hospital in the country. In charge of the hospital was Rufus Cole, a recognised expert in the management of pneumonia.

One effect of the First World War in the United States even before it had joined in the fighting, was that resources were directed away from the scientific projects including Kleiner's work to what the authorities at the Institute considered more important to the war effort. The possibility of infectious disease, as had happened during the Spanish American War, was fresh in their minds.

The American government began drafting young men to go to war, which increased the size of the US military troops from 150,000 to the eventual number in excess of 4 million. Such a large number, housed in cramped quarters came with its own problems, namely, infectious disease. Memories of this as a cause of the death of thousands of troops during the Spanish American war haunted the authorities.

The Rockefeller Institute director Flexner directed the resources of the institution almost in its entirety to the war effort. It's scientists were directed to the development of antisera for treating infectious diseases like meningitis, dysentery and pneumonia. The Institute was a now „war demonstration hospital".

Nearly all its physicians travelled to different camps to supervise the treatment of infectious disease.

Kleiner was increasingly isolated from the war effort because his training and research had nothing to contribute to the needs produced by the conflict.

In 1917 largely through Flexner's suggestion, the Rockefeller Institute in its entirety was incorporated as an auxiliary post of the US army and, in the same year, Flexner terminated Kleiner's employment at the Rockefeller Institute.

Kleiner returned to Yale to teach the classes which had been taught by Mendel before he had been called up for war service.

When armistice was declared in November 1918, Kleiner expected to return to the Rockefeller and resume his research, but Flexner's plans did not include this because according to him the young scientist's

> *"work is not essential to the Institute's war program. I believe it would be well for Kleiner to go into teaching, and this may be the time to make the change. He is not a man the Institute wishes to attach itself to permanently".*

Towards the end of 1918, Kleiner was told that his term at the Institute would end by June 1919. At no point did Flexner engage in any discussion on Kleiner's research or its importance in the treatment of the thousands of patients with diabetes.

In the fall of 1919, Kleiner submitted his final paper on diabetes research as a single author.

26

END OF THE ODYSSEY

The lucid exposition of Kleiner's work as presented by Friedman made me imagine the Rockefeller professor in a barrister's gown and, out of respect for a tradition dating back to the late 1600s, donning the horsehair wig to complete the outfit before beginning his summing up.

Referring to Kleiner's final article Friedman said, "it was an extraordinary piece of work – a masterpiece, even", before continuing.

"At a time when most scientific papers reported their data through anecdotes in a way that would be regarded as unconvincing, or even slapdash today, Kleiner showed, by precise evidentiary standards, and in a large group of animals, that the pancreas, (but not other tissues) made a hormone that regulated blood glucose. And rather than dwell on this finding answered the esoteric question of why glucose was retained in the blood of diabetics, Kleiner now went directly to the core of the medical problem with a focus not evident in his earlier papers. He repeatedly emphasised the clinical implications of his findings, writing that they "suggest a possible therapeutic application," and also speculated on whether an extract of the pancreas from another species would have the same effect, thus predicting the use of extracts prepared from animals (cows and later, pigs in the case of the Canadian team of Banting and Best). Kleiner closed by writing that the "effective agent or agents, their purification, concentration, and identification are suggested as promising fields for further work.

Indeed, they were".

When I read this, I thought that the details Friedman had provided summed up Kleiner's contributions and he would leave it there.

But I was wrong.

The highly regarded current researcher was just warming up.

Couched in a longer sentence he asked a blunt, one-word question.

"Why?"

If Flexner was the reason for Kleiner's research grinding to a halt, Friedman's is the obvious question. Why would Flexner, who was recognised as a shrewd judge of talent and good sense, fail to appreciate the historic discovery that was within Kleiner's, and the Institute's, reach?

Friedman then presented a balanced and reasoned opinion.

He began slowly, gently.

Kleiner was a young scientist. His work which was being carried out at the Rockefeller during World War II was an important research project on the cause of diabetes.

Friedman acknowledged, and agreed with, the importance of the emphasis placed by Flexner, and the United States Army physician William Gorgas, on the need to improve and maintain the health care of the US troops by controlling and treating infectious disease.

He pointed out that the treatment of Kleiner

"presupposes that we know what will be important in the future. Infectious disease was the priority for Flexner and it is likely that he would have been shocked to learn that diabetes, although perhaps a boutique illness in his day, has since become a massive worldwide public health crisis."

(Italics by the writer.)

Then, perhaps feeling that he had gone in too hard on an absent older colleague from an earlier time, Friedman relented, saying

"Still, Flexner's intense focus on the catastrophe (ie World War I) unfolding in front of him is easy to understand, and while great discoveries are obvious in hindsight, it is considerably more difficult to discern one in the making. Identifying the person who will make that kind of discovery can be similarly difficult. The personal traits required for success in science are highly varied…

Some are intense and outwardly confident, like Flexner, while others are more timid and easier to overlook, like Kleiner. Friedman had succeeded in tracking down Kleiner's two grandsons one of whom remembered his grandfather as "the mildest man in the world."

Friedman then proposed that another reason which contributed to denying Kleiner the distinction and fame which otherwise may have been his was his quiet and self effacing personality.

As far as is known, Kleiner did not react to, let alone resist Flexner's lack of interest in his work after the end of the war.

Stopping short of invoking the researcher's personality as being any more than a minor contributory factor, Friedman noted the lack of support the young scientist had received from Flexner. Perhaps as a young researcher himself looking at an event with hindsight, he felt that he had said enough and left the issue as a challenge for the reader.

Kleiner's final paper on the subject of diabetes appeared in 1919. He described a hormone produced by the pancreas which regulated glucose and suggested extraction from other animals could be used to check blood sugar levels. He did not proceed any further with research on diabetes after this.

However, he remained interested in developments associated with insulin as evidenced by his attendance at the meeting of the American Physiological Society in New Haven in 1921 where

Frederick Banting and James Macleod had presented the findings of research carried out at the University of Toronto.

Their findings were published in a paper in February 1922, in which they stated that pancreatic extracts

> *"do have a reducing effect on blood sugar, thus confirming Kleiner."*

(Italics by the writer).

Bliss's book does not mention Kleiner's presence at the New Haven meeting let alone any mention of his work which was acknowledged in the paper mentioned above. Kleiner was not the type to jump up and speak of his own work especially in a meeting which was attended by many who would not have known him.

Commenting on his work on insulin many years later, Kleiner was typically restrained. He said "… the First World War had come about and interfered… '' with his pursuit of the glucose-regulating hormone".

After reading Friedman's article and his reflections on Kleiner's personality, I was reminded of comments made by a young "current" scientist on some of the personal and professional characteristics which are helpful in the challenging and competitive fields of scientific research.

Scientia Professor Michelle Simmons, FRS who won the 2021 Bakerian Medal and Lecture and works at University of New South Wales in Sydney said,

> *"We all have our feelings and prejudices. Even with the most careful adherence to the scientific method, it's difficult to see the world as it truly is. One has to be systematic, and observant of details. This takes a certain amount of bloody-mindedness and grit."*
>
> (Italics by the writer).

Kleiner's last employment was at the New York Homeopathic College where he spent the rest of his professional life. He did not engage in any further research on insulin. Israel Kleiner died in 1966.

27

INSULIN RESEARCHERS WHOSE FINDINGS PRECEDED BANTING'S

Several claims of having discovered insulin before the Toronto team have been aired. These are discussed below. Some but not all of these claims were made not after the announcement of the discovery in the medical literature, but after the Nobel Prize had been awarded to Banting and Macleod.

The Nobel committee stipulates that it does not change its decision after the prize has been presented.

An examination of the literature clearly demonstrates that well before the Toronto team of Frederick Banting and Best had started on the project which ultimately led to the discovery of insulin, workers on both sides of the Atlantic had been involved in research on the pancreas, particularly in the late 1800s and the early 1900s.

Included in the examples of reports preceding Banting's and Best's experiments is the work of the Frenchman Eugene Gley perhaps the most dramatic and intriguing account of all.

Eugene Gley (1857–1930).

Eugene Gley was born into an academic family, his father being a professor of Latin. Gley started medical studies at the University of Montpellier but most of his life was spent in Paris, where a special Chair was created for him to continue his studies in physiology.

Gley occupied the Chair of General Biology at the College de France from 1908 to the end of his life in 1930.

Impressed by the hypothesis of his fellow countryman Gustave-Eduard Laguesse (1861–1927) which held that the secretion/s of the Islets of Langerhans prevented the loss of glucose in the urine, Gley tested it by administering such an extract to dogs made diabetic by removal of the pancreas. He noted that not only was there less sugar in the urine specimens of the animals but that the animals were less troubled by thirst and frequent passage of urine.

Gley went further to determine if the results he had obtained were entirely due to the effects of the islets of Langerhans. He isolated the tissue of the islets from which he prepared an extract which was injected into the diabetic dogs. Once again, the extract significantly reduced the amount of sugar being lost in the urine.

Gley's experiments on diabetic dogs were essentially the same as those carried out by Frederick Banting in Toronto, 25 years later.

The Gley Incident. An Historic Folly ?

After completing his experiments Gley wrote a report, sealed it in an envelope and handed it to the "Societe Francaise de Biologie" in 1905, with a recommendation that the envelope be opened only upon his request.

Gley did not repeat his experiments on the pancreas but on hearing of Frederick Banting's experiments in 1921, he gave the order to open the envelope having realised that he had actually discovered insulin several years earlier without realising it.

In addition to his impressive scientific credentials, Gley was also known for exercising restraint verging on reluctance to draw conclusions from the results of his scientific work prematurely.

This character trait in the French scientist may have played an important part in the insulin story and one which, as related above, may well have haunted the publicity-shy researcher in the twilight years of his distinguished career.

He had made the request at the meeting of the society held on December 23, 1922 after hearing the news of the discovery in Toronto.

Gley made no claim to have discovered insulin, and indeed sent a congratulatory note to Macleod for simplifying his (Gley's) method.

Gley died in 1930.

The Nobel Foundation (2015) Nomination Database reveals that in 1921, 1925, 1926, 1928 and 1931 Gley received fifty-one nominations for the Nobel Prize. In 1921 alone, there were 11 nominations for him. Whether these were related to the reports of the discovery of insulin in Toronto is unclear. However, like several other luminaries in the insulin story, including Oskar Minkowski and Claude Bernard, Gley did not win the Nobel Prize.

An Earlier French Contribution to the Cause of Diabetes.

Etienne Lancereux (1829–1910), is known for his contributions in the early years of the European scholars' attempts to understand diabetes.

After obtaining his doctorate in 1862, Lancereux worked in various various hospitals conducting research in order to find the organ responsible for diabetes.

In 1877 he published a paper which contained the term "diabete pancreatique" which he had coined because he believed that the cause of diabetes was located in the pancreas. This was later confirmed by the experiments of Minkowski and von Mering in 1889.

Lancereaux based his opinions on clinical studies as well as autopsies on patients with diabetes.

Together with Apollinaire Bouchardat he had made the original observation that diabetes existed in two forms, namely diabetes of the thin (diabete maigre), and diabetes of the fat (diabete gras).

In addition to classifying the condition into the two groups the French physician had also commented that the thin diabetic patient had a poorer outlook with early death as compared with the Type 2 variety which stood a better chance of a long life. Both these findings were dramatically illustrated in the tragic plight of children who contracted the condition in the years before the discovery of insulin.

The two forms are now more commonly referred to as Type 1 and Type 2 diabetes respectively.

From the point of view of the history of early research on diabetes in Europe, it is interesting that one of Lancereaux's students was Nicolas Paulescu (1869–1931) whose seminal contributions to the discovery of insulin have been detailed earlier in this account.

Lydia Maria Adams De Witt (1859–1928).

De Witt had graduated in Medicine from Michigan University in 1886 and had initially served in the pathology department there. Most of her working life was spent at the University of Chicago from 1912 to1926.

Less well known is De Witt's work during the early years of her interest in the pancreas.

In 1906, experimenting with cats she demonstrated that tying off the pancreatic duct destroyed most of the pancreas.

When she prepared an extract from the remnant, which included the islets of Langerhans, she showed that there was a beneficial effect on diabetes although the effect was said to be minor, presumably as shown by only a small reduction in the level of glucose in the blood or the loss of it in the urine of the experimental cats.

Ernest Lyman Scott (1877–1966).

Ernest Scott probably carried out the earliest logical and successful series of experiments which showed that an extract he had prepared from the pancreas relieved the major abnormalities in diabetes namely, increased blood sugar level and loss of sugar in the urine. These results were published in the *American Journal of Physiology* in 1912.

Unfortunately, Scott's work on insulin was reported in an article written several years after he had done the work. It has remained a subject of controversy on the thorny topic of *scientific priority* of significant discoveries relating to insulin and diabetes.

The story relates to Scott's early postgraduate career. Born in Kinsman, Ohio Scott went to Ohio Wesleyan University and graduated with B.S.in 1902. He then went to the University of Chicago and received his MS in 1911.

It was during his time in Chicago that he did his work on insulin. The Head of the Department of Physiology was Anton Carlson.

Anton Julius Carlson (1875–1956) was of Swedish extraction. He was a respected researcher and had been in charge of the administration of the department for some years when Scott joined him. The capable student carried out the work on the isolation of the pancreatic extract with little if any input by Carlson. However, as a student working towards a masters degree, Scott, like any other student was at least theoretically working under the guidance of the head namely, Carlson. However, much of his work was done independently of any meaningful input from Carlson.

Scott's thesis written in 1911 included details of the preparation of an extract which benefited experimental diabetic dogs.

He only stayed in Chicago in 1911 and 1912 before moving from there to the University of Kansas briefly, and then to Columbia University where he spent the rest of his life except for war service during World War I with the American expeditionary Force in France.

At Columbia he continued his work on glucose and developed tests for measuring blood glucose as a method of identifying diabetes.

When Scott left Chicago, he had left his thesis with Carlson. Carlson published a version of Scott's thesis (in Scott's name) in 1912 in the *American Journal of Physiology*. Carlson, it is said, had largely edited Scott's contribution out of the experiments.

Scott later categorically denied any authorship of the article which Carlson had written based on his young associate's work. Scott claimed that Carlson had made significant changes with which Scott disagreed. The thesis in its original form was published in 1966.

After the award of the Nobel Prize, Scott wrote to congratulate Banting as a "logical recipient" but noted that "the discovery of the curative power of insulin has been open from January 1912, to anyone who cared to repeat and extend my work."

According to Michael Bliss as recorded in his book *The Discovery of Insulin*, Scott was present at the meeting at Yale University, New Haven on December 30, 1920. After the meeting, Scott had walked back to the hotel with Macleod and had told him about his work which had been done in 1911. He had followed up on his discussion by sending Macleod the details of his extraction method, suggesting that employing his method, might avoid the adverse reactions which had troubled the Toronto team. However Scott admitted that his method had never been put to the "severe trials" Banting's team was experiencing in Toronto.

Scott's wife, Aleita Hopping Scott, a physiologist with a PhD in the subject was convinced that her husband had been denied the credit due to him. In 1972 she wrote a book, *Great Scott. Ernest Lyman Scott's Work With Insulin in 1911.*

George Ludwig Zuelzer (1870–1949).

In 1908 Zuelzer, an internist in Berlin, demonstrated the beneficial effect of injecting pancreatic extracts in a dying diabetic patient. However the beneficial effect was short-lived and Zuelzer was unable to prepare sufficient amounts of the extract in time to save the patient's life…

When the Nobel prize was awarded to Banting and Macleod, Zuelzer demanded that he be considered the discoverer of insulin. He remained vocal in his later years when he migrated from his native Germany to the United States.

Michael Bliss in his book on the discovery of insulin related the story of the German scientist visiting Charles Best in Toronto and insisting on being recognised as the person who had discovered the hormone.

Zuelzer died in a facility for the aged in New York in 1952.

By 1912, several scholars, including the Italians Massaglia and Zannini, (ref.Levene), were satisfied that the destruction of the part of the pancreas which is involved in digestion did not cause diabetes, whereas destroying the islets of Langerhans did.

Nicolae Constantin Paulescu (1869–1931).

Paulescu, from a wealthy aristocratic Rumanian family had studied in medicine in Paris under Ettienne Lancereaux, a respected physician and one of the early authorities on diabetes had made significant contributions on diabetes in the French medical literature long before Paulesco joined him in Paris in 1888.

Paulesco's interest in diabetes was undoubtedly begun through the long-standing interest of his professor in the condition. It was not surprising that the gifted medical student who graduated with a Doctorate in Medicine in 1897, continued with research into the condition when he returned to Romania in 1900.

He quickly rose to become the Head of the Department of Physiology at the University of Bucharest Medical School.

Paulesco also held a permanent position as Professor of Clinical Medicine at the St Vincent de Paul in hospital in Bucharest until his death in 1931.

His research included studying the changes in the blood of patients with diabetes.

Paulescu started his experiments on dogs in Bucharest in 1916 but stopped due to WW1. Later he returned to complete his research in 1920–1921.

In 1916 he had succeeded in preparing pancreatic extracts from dogs' pancreases. Injecting these extracts into experimental animals (dogs), he had found that the level of blood sugar fell as did the amount of sugar being lost in the urine.

In 1921, eight months before Banting's first publication in February 1922, Paulesco published his results in French journals.

He called the new hormone *pancreine* and, believing that it would be an important element in the treatment of diabetes, took out a patent on it.

Unfortunately, the results of giving pancreine to diabetic subjects did not produce consistent results.

Regardless of the inconsistencies in the use of his product, there has been strong support for Paulescu being entitled to the Nobel Prize because his work preceded the experiments carried out in Toronto.

Paulesco's methods for preparing the extract were similar to those used by Israel Kleiner who had published his work in the *Journal of Biological Chemistry* in 1919. Paulesco, on the other hand, had chosen a less widely known publication which had a smaller circulation. The details of his experiments and their results appeared in the August 1921 issue of *Archives Internationales de Physiologie* in Belgium. He had submitted the paper on 22nd of June,1921.

Paulesco had also written a book *New Insights Into Experimental Diabetes* (University of Paris, 1897–1901).

His experiments provided convincing evidence that his extract, which he called *pancreine*, lowered the level of blood glucose in diabetic animals.

Unfortunately, like the Toronto workers, he had difficulty in producing the extract in adequate quantities for use in the large number of patients who were in urgent need of treatment. Neither could Paulesco resolve the problems of purification which Banting and Macleod had achieved with the help of the biochemist Collip and later through their association with the chemist George Walden of the Lilly Company.

Nicolae Paulescu's name was largely promoted by European scientists and physicians who noted the interruption of the war as the reason for his failure to publish his findings, which he had made before the discovery in Toronto.

In terms of priority, it is pertinent to note that Paulesco had prepared pancreatic extracts in 1916 when he had tested it in dogs while Israel Kleiner had tested pancreatic extracts in his dogs a year earlier in 1915.

The German scientist Giorg Zuelzer had done so even earlier in 1906.

All three extracts prepared and tested in living subjects by Zuelzer, Kleiner and Paulesco had caused side-effects either in dogs or in humans. So for that matter, had the extract prepared by Banting's team.

However, only Banting had persisted with improving the extract to the point of it being suitable for use in patients with diabetes.

Of all the researchers before the work in Toronto only Banting had stayed the course till insulin was produced commercially in the quantities needed to treat the large numbers of patients with diabetes.

The most gracious response of one of the many men and women engaged in the pursuit of insulin who could claim priority in its discovery, came from Oskar Minkowski who said, "I too share with Doctor Zuelzer, the regret that I did *not* discover insulin."

The role of Carlson as well as Flexner, together with the well documented confrontations between Banting and the Ontario-born Scotsman, Duncan Graham, all highlight the influence – and challenge – of "managers" including administrators and bureaucrats in the wider field of administration.

28

THE NOBEL CONTROVERSY IN TORONTO. A POSTSCRIPT

Public outpouring of joy and goodwill on and celebrations of the discovery of insulin were far less sustained than the controversy which has dogged the 1923 Nobel award for the entire 100 years since that event.

Allotting the credit for the discovery to different members of the team began almost as soon as the discovery had been made. Nearly everyone, qualified or otherwise, ranging from hospital personnel to the doctors, young and old, had an opinion on the person responsible for the breakthrough.

Nor was the practice restricted to Toronto. In the Best family archives, there is mention of differing opinions in the medical circles in England at the time of the discovery on whether Banting or Macleod was the more deserving of the Nobel Prize. The older members of the English medical establishment favoured Macleod as the more deserving while the younger ones were for Banting. Another claimed that the discovery of insulin was entirely attributable to the efforts of two natives of Scotland because Macleod, educated in Aberdeen was a Scotsman, as was Duncan Graham, the bureaucrat who had barred Banting from the early trials of the insulin extract prepared by Banting and Best, and later by Collip.

Given the claims and opinions of the English and Scottish individuals in this controversy it is perhaps not mischievous to include an Irish contribution.

Here I borrow from the talented Mr. Patrick Redden Keefe who spoke of a new term in his book *Say Nothing* (William Collins, 2018).

It is *whataboutery.*

The term came into use in Ireland during discussions on the contribution by different individuals to a given incident or aspect of the Troubles, such as acts of betrayal.

The same could be said about the varying opinions on who should have been awarded the Nobel prize as is still seen in many articles and books more than 100 years after the event. There are varying opinions on the merit or otherwise of Banting versus another individual as being more deserving. "What about Paulescu?" and "what about Zuelzer ?" Then, what about Banting's much publicised choice of his helper Charles Best? *whatabout… whatabout* ......etc.

As is often the way with publicity, new headlines soon replaced both insulin and Banting, at least in the short term. However, the issue of priority relating to the discovery was to be re-visited repeatedly over the years and persists to this day.

In some scientific circles widespread differences of opinion on the appropriateness of the Nobel Prize having been given to Frederick Banting still attract vigorous debate.

Banting's attack on James Macleod was based on the young man's conviction that Macleod had appropriated the credit for the discovery which Banting believed belonged to him and his student helper, Charles Best. From this it followed that the Nobel Prize awarded to Banting should not have been shared with Macleod. Banting's reaction to the award was to share half of his monetary reward with Best. This was followed by Macleod giving part of his share to Collip who had been instrumental in achieving the critical breakthrough by finding a method of preparing an extract pure enough to be tried on a human patient.

Each of the four members of the Toronto team reacted differently to the reward received for the discovery.

Banting maintained the rage to the end of his life. Collip did not enter into the discussion other than saying that he would let the scientific publications speak for themselves.

Macleod, after leaving Toronto in 1928, never made any comment of note on the Nobel award. Best never reconciled himself to not receiving a share of the prize.

Best's Reaction to not Receiving the Nobel Prize.

Best never reconciled himself to the decision of the Nobel Committee which, according to the rules of the award, is empowered to make the decision based on the nominations received. Charles Best had not received a single nomination and therefore was not considered for the award. Furthermore, apart from Banting, he had few supporters who considered him as being worthy of that degree of recognition.

The highly respected American physiologist Francis Gano Benedict (1870–1957) in his nomination of Banting had specified that in his opinion there was none other worthy of sharing the award. A comment from another physician at the time was less kind, comparing Best's role to that of a young apprentice working in a mechanic's shop assigned "the task of handing the spanner to the mechanic."

According to the personal records contained in the family archives and published by his son Henry Bruce Macleod Best in the excellent biography of his parents, *Margaret and Charlie The Personal Story of Dr. Charles Best, the Co - Discoverer of Insulin* published in 2003, Charles Best appears to have made it clear that he should have received equal recognition with Banting.

Best remained in Toronto for the rest of his working life. He was always the first "port of call" when it came to speaking on the subject of insulin in the years following it's discovery.

He travelled to various parts of the world, including Australia, where he was received with ceremony and accorded recognition and respect, even adulation.

On one occasion when describing their trip to Sweden – his wife always accompanied him – he commented, in his family records, on the praise and recognition he was given, then added words to the effect that some of this may have been to make up for not having giving him the Nobel Prize.

In his later years one of the few public accounts of the discovery which were documented in detail were by Best himself. They are contained in a recording which has been preserved by the London branch of the Osler Society. The Society had invited Best to deliver the Osler Oration in London in 1957 on the 36th anniversary of the discovery. Best was 58 years old. After checking with the organisers that the lecture was not going to be published, Best was expansive in his description of the time spent on discovering insulin.

Listening to the recording, it is difficult to distinguish Best's contributions from those of Banting. There was no mention of the time spent by Banting in persuading Macleod to agree to Banting's ideas for isolating insulin or the fact that Best was seconded to Banting as a helper during Best's summer holidays from his Science course. (The decision for Best to assist Banting had been decided on a coin toss).

Collip and Macleod were barely mentioned in Best's lecture.

In 2003 Charles Best's second son Henry Best (1937–2006), a retired historian, wrote a book *Margaret and Charlie, The Personal Story of Dr Charles Best, the Co-Discoverer of Insulin.*

The bulk of the material contained in this well-written account of his parents' lives was derived from the voluminous records of letters, notes and diaries of both Charles Best and his wife Margaret Mahon Best.

In 1961, nearly 40 years after the Nobel award to Banting and Macleod, Henry Best interviewed Professor Rolf Luft who, at that time, was the secretary of the Nobel Committee. What Henry Best may not have known is that Rolf Luft had a special interest in diabetes and in fact at that time was the secretary of the much respected International Diabetes Federation (IDF).

My own interest in diabetes and membership of the IDF had given me several opportunities to talk to Dr Luft, although we never discussed the issue of Best's story and the 1923 Nobel Prize.

Henry Best's book quoted Luft's measured – some might say diplomatic – response.

"I can say that, with reservations, I think that it might have been fair to give the prize to Banting, Best and Paulesco."

Luft was nothing if not a consummate medical diplomat.

Speculations on Reasons for Banting's Success.

Scholars and scientists had pursued diabetes for centuries. Physicians had described it in ancient times. Many of these men and women justifiably occupy prominent positions in the history of medical research. Yet it was a young medical graduate with virtually no experience in medical research who succeeded in solving one of the great modern medical mysteries.

Scepticism is regarded by some as part of human nature. It may manifest itself in many ways as happened following the discovery of insulin by a little-known researcher in a university in one of the British colonies, Canada. Toronto was hardly considered a "seat of learning" especially in the English-speaking world. The cream of English (medical) intelligentsia resided in the recognised and premier centres of learning like Oxford and Cambridge. After all, the much admired William Osler, the American – actually a Canadian by birth – had required little persuasion to move from his position as Professor of Medicine of Johns Hopkins Hospital in Baltimore, USA, when offered the Regius Professorship in Medicine at Oxford University in 1904.

The scepticism of the English following the discovery of insulin by Banting manifested itself in the sending of two senior academics and researchers, Henry Dale and Harold Dudley to Toronto to see the Canadians as well as their experiments and laboratories for themselves.

To be fair, Dale had been quick to acknowledge the success of Banting's research. Reporting back to his associates in London Dale had said, "We arrived in Toronto towards the end of September and the evidence put before us carried immediate conviction that a genuine discovery of great potential importance had been made.

Professor James J.R. Macleod had organised a team of workers to reinforce the activities of the original discoverers in work directed to the improvement of methods for estimating the amount of insulin present in extracts, and to the production of purer preparations in a higher yield. The practical production was, indeed still is, in its infancy."

The account errs in the essential question of initiating the project which was attributed by Dale to Macleod whereas the undisputed fact is that the exercise in its entirety was initiated by Banting.

Similarly, two respected German physicians namely, Karl von Noorden, a specialist in diabetes and the highly regarded Bernhard Naunyn, both doubted the importance of the discovery made in Toronto. Naunyn considered the reports of Banting's findings an example of "American exaggeration."

Stories abound of the transformation of lives through the use of insulin in the treatment of diabetes around the world. Some of them have been recounted in this work.

29

BANTING'S (UNSPOKEN AND UNWRITTEN) ANSWER TO THE PRIORITY RULE

"Our main business in life is not to see what lies dimly at a distance, but to do what lies clearly at hand."
Thomas Carlyle.

The epigram, which William Osler adopted as his personal motto and which he quoted to his students throughout his life, may well apply to the urgent need for insulin for treating patients with diabetes at the time of its pursuit and the celebrated discovery by Frederick Banting.

The "Bench to the Bedside" test in the Insulin Story.

There is no record of Banting's response to questions of priority in the discovery of insulin other than his much publicised quarrel with Macleod.

Apart from his concern and compassion, which in much of the literature on the subject of the discovery of insulin, has taken second place to his belligerence in dealing with Macleod, there is also the question of priorities, not in recording or publishing experiments but of getting supplies of insulin to the patient. This has often been referred to as the "bench to the bedside rule." It gets little emphasis in most articles in the literature, including the medical journals.

The patients who until then were living each day with the very real possibility of death hanging over their heads numbered in the thousands around the world.

The one significant difference between those who recorded the results of their experiments in various journals before Banting and Best, is that only the Toronto group delivered the product developed in their laboratory to the patient. Furthermore, in the Toronto group, the driving force from the beginning of the pursuit to locate, then isolate prior to refining the extract and making it suitable for injecting into the patient with diabetes was Fred Banting.

Only Banting.

No one else.

It must be remembered that Banting was the only practising doctor in the group.

His unshakeable priority of providing insulin to patients suffering from diabetes separates him from the many other dedicated researchers and scientists engaged in the pursuit of the elusive extract.

Anecdotal reports of his contact with the parents of children afflicted with the life-threatening disorder appeared repeatedly in my reading of the history of diabetes at that time.

I was sent a copy of an article in the Medical Journal of Australia by Professor Milton Roxanas which told the story of a five-year-old girl whose father had written to Banting even before the extract had been prepared. Banting had written back to him, urging and encouraging the very concerned and frightened parent to keep to the diet and reassuring him that they were in the final stages of producing an effective extract. When the extract was dispatched (by sea) the article described the father not waiting for the ship that was carrying the extract to berth at the terminal near the Sydney Harbour Bridge but getting into a speedboat and going aboard the vessel which was waiting in the harbour before berthing. The five-year-old girl, six by the time she got her first injection of insulin, was Australia's first recipient of the magic potion. The story of Phyllis Lush has been recounted earlier.

The same article also detailed the efforts of an Adelaide professor, T.P. Robertson who had been in Toronto at the time of the discovery of insulin, and who later was instrumental in getting supplies of the hormone to Adelaide.

Banting's insistence on developing insulin to the stage where it could be injected into the patient is in sharp contrast with the experiments of the researchers described below. Admittedly, some of them were foiled by circumstances beyond their control. The disruption caused by World War I has been described above through the tragic circumstances of Israel Kleiner's research.

There are also accounts of Banting writing back to the parents and doctors especially of children who were suffering from diabetes when the first reports of the isolation of insulin in Toronto were published in Canadian, American and English newspapers. Therefore, in terms of a meaningful connection with the patients and their relatives, Banting had progressed further than the any of the other researchers.

Yet the controversy over the credit for discovering insulin and awarding the Nobel Prize to Banting has continued. As recently as 2012, on the 90th anniversary of the discovery, a review article in a prestigious scientific journal recorded the differing views of several respected medical authorities on the appropriateness or otherwise of awarding of the Nobel Prize to Banting and Macleod. Several of the contributors noted the experiments on insulin (as detailed in this work) which had been carried out before the team of Banting, Best, Macleod and Collip had done their work in Toronto.

The emphasis, once again, was on the individual or the team who/which had achieved the goal and published the results *first*, the so-called "Priority Rule" rule in scientific publications.

30

THE LATER LIVES OF THE TORONTO RESEARCHERS

After the discovery of insulin the four men involved in the exercise went their separate ways.

Sir Frederick Grant Banting.

Banting was feted in Canada throughout his life. He was in constant demand to attend public and institutional functions ranging from opening national exhibits to giving lectures. He was given a lifelong appointment at the University. He had also resumed his artistic activities which had begun with oil painting during the lean times in the early years of his attempt at general practice. Banting did not engage in any serious research, even though he maintained his appointment at Toronto University.

His application to enlist for active duty as an Army Medical Officer in World War II (1939–1945), was denied given his national prominence but he was persuaded to accept a more senior position as chairman of a medical research committee involved in Canada's war time activities.

On February 20, he boarded a Hudson bomber in Gander, Newfoundland bound for England. Shortly after takeoff, the aircraft stalled, possibly due to the formation of ice in a part of the engine. Banting survived the crash, was rescued and transferred to hospital, but died shortly afterwards. He was 49.

Thus ended the life of the flawed, remarkable, and very human individual who alone thought, actually dreamt of, then pursued the hitherto elusive hormone to its discovery. Furthermore, undistracted by adulation, controversy and other obstacles he stayed the course until he could bring the hormone to those who most needed it – the children, men and women who until that time had faced imminent death from diabetes.

In completing this last essential step of delivering insulin to suffering humanity, Banting rightfully earned pride of place in the insulin story. This, more than any other consideration, including the Priority Rule for research publications, distinguishes Banting the inexperienced researcher from other respected authorities of his time as well the earlier scientists and scholars who had made important contributions to the knowledge of insulin before the Toronto experiments.

Charles Best.

Best remained in Toronto for the rest of his professional life, but enjoyed the fruits of the discovery of insulin by being in constant demand for giving lectures on the subject and being honoured internationally especially during various anniversaries, not only of the discovery of insulin but other important dates in the calendar of diabetes. He travelled extensively throughout the world invariably referred to as "the discoverer of insulin." Ignoring the condition of being nominated before being considered for the award by the Nobel Committee, Best never accepted its decision not to give him the prize.

He succeeded James Macleod as Head of the Department of Physiology at the University of Toronto, when Macleod returned to Scotland upon completion of his tenure. Macleod himself had nominated the 29-year-old whom he had taught but who had no experience in administration. Best also served as Research Director of Connaught Laboratories.

He remained at Toronto University for the rest of his working life.

Best died of a ruptured aorta at the age of 79 on 31 March 1978.

James Macleod.

James Macleod returned to his native Scotland in 1928 as the Regius Professor at the University of Aberdeen, his alma mater. He was highly regarded at home but lived largely out of the limelight. In 1935, seven years after his return to Scotland, Macleod died in his sleep from complications of severe arthritis. He was 59 years old.

Macleod never spoke publicly about the discovery of insulin.

James Collip who was only 27 at the time of the saga of the discovery of insulin in Toronto where his important contribution has never been in question, returned to his previous position in early 1922.

He devoted his entire life to medical research, mostly at McGill University.

Collip isolated several hormones, including "Premarin" a hormone which became one of the highest selling pharmaceutical products in the world. He was highly respected as the leader of research in Canada.

Collip did not seem embittered by not sharing the Nobel Prize.

His usual answer to question on priority of the discovery of insulin was that he was "happy to let the insulin story stand on the publications by the group who collaborated in 1921–1922."

In later years Collip had befriended Frederick Banting. They had seen each other just before Banting's final journey which ended in the tragedy of the fatal plane crash. On what turned out to be the final evening of his life, Banting had gone to visit Collip. It was bitterly cold and Collip noticed that Banting, being his usual disorganised self, did not have any gloves. He gave his sheepskin gloves to Banting to wear on the journey. This was the ill-fated journey which ended in the tragedy of Banting's death in the plane crash in Newfoundland.

So ends the story of the discovery of insulin just over 100 years ago but the remarkable transformation of the lives of millions by the discovery holds its place in the history of science and is ranked by some as the greatest medical discovery in history.

A Footnote.

William Banting, Queen Victoria's Undertaker.

There are no facts to link an Englishman, William Banting (1796–1878), to the better known Frederick Banting, who discovered insulin. However, there may be a connection given the fact that the Bantings of Toronto originally came from Britain.

There are interesting connections between the English Banting and diabetes.

William Banting was the head of one of the leading firms of funeral directors (yes, funeral directors) in Britain. The firm had conducted the funerals of English monarchs starting with King George the Third in 1820 through to Queen Victoria in 1901 and King Edward the Seventh in 1910.

William Banting's connection with diabetes may lie in the fact that he carried a weight of 202 pounds for his height of 5'7" and was advised by the physician William Harvey to lose weight by using the method of limiting the intake of carbohydrates "especially starch of sugary nature." Harvey had learned of this type of diet to be of benefit in the treatment of diabetes because he had attended lectures in Paris by the eminent French physiologist and physician Claude Bernard whose contributions to diabetes are mentioned more than once in this account.

William Banting also wrote a booklet, called *Letter on Corpulence, Addressed to the Public*, which was published in 1863 and detailed limiting starchy and sweet foods.

Interestingly, he also wrote of his unsuccessful attempts through fasting, use of spas and various exercise programs recommended by different medical experts. Then, stating what might get present-day practitioners into some difficulty with governing bodies, he stated "my kind and valued medical advisor is not a doctor for obesity, but stands on the pinnacle of fame in the treatment of another malady, which, as he well knows, is frequently induced by corpulence." One assumes that the condition referred to was diabetes.

William Banting's booklet turned out to be a "best seller" the profits from which he donated to charity. Although he had published the account at his own expense, the third and later editions were published by a London publisher and were still in print in the early 2000s.

Some diets described as the Banting diet, contrary to popular belief, are based on the William Banting booklet, not his more illustrious namesake of the insulin fame.

31

BANTING'S GREATEST ACHIEVEMENT

The controversy, especially over the awarding of the Nobel prize for the discovery of insulin has, to some extent, overshadowed the importance of the discovery in the bigger picture of the treatment of diabetes.

It is in this area that Banting is without equal among those who pursued the hormone. True, that World War I interfered with the research of other workers, including Kleiner and Paulesco, but the fact remains that only Banting remained at the helm after discovering insulin until he was able to deliver supplies of the lifesaving medicine to patients directly or through their doctors.

Banting had also encountered interference and obstruction, as well as discouragement verging on ridicule by bureaucrats. World War I had also impacted his progress through medical school and military service.

His battles with bureaucrats are described in detail in the book by Bliss which contains accounts of the hurdles faced by Banting in getting the insulin extract tested on patients in the hospital in Toronto. Duncan Graham, although born in Ontario, was proud of his Scottish heritage and had sided with the scotsman Macleod in the quarrels between Banting and the professor. He had used his authority to bar Banting from the ward when the extract prepared by the team of Banting, Best, and Collip was injected into a patient.

It is important not to lose sight of the fact that from the early earliest stages of embarking on the search for insulin which dated back to October 31, 1920, Banting had always considered the real test of his work to be the effect of the extract on a human diabetic. Even though barred from entering the ward, Banting and Best had stayed outside in the corridor while the extract they had prepared was being injected into a patient not as Banting had hoped, by him but by an intern in the medical team of Walter Campbell, the physician who was the head of that particular unit in Toronto Hospital.

So, unlike the mild mannered Israel Kleiner as well as the scholarly Frenchman Gley and the combative German Zuelzer, only Banting through dogged determination, even bloody-mindedness, had stayed the course until he had succeeded in producing an extract of *an acceptable quality and quantity* to witness its injection into patients suffering from diabetes.

However, even discovering insulin, then proving that it reduced the level of glucose in the blood would have been of little value had not the project continued to the point of commercial manufacture.

In this area also Banting had no equal among the other workers, who with varying degrees of success had worked on the project of discovering or isolating insulin.

The less attractive aspects of Banting's personality have been described, dissected and repeated in many publications, including recent ones. There have been criticisms of the methods he used in the laboratory, often judged by today's standards and by workers who have had the advantage of better training and mentoring, to say nothing of accessibility to modern technologies.

Hindsight is a valuable tool but should it not take into account the conditions prevailing at the time of a given event, in this case, the discovery of insulin in the 1920s ?

It is surprising that few, if any of the dissenting submissions on the subject of credit for the discovery of insulin recognised the essential difference between Banting and the others including members of Banting's own team.

It is likely that Banting himself was not aware of the various conventions such as the priority rule in reporting new findings in scientific journals as was followed especially by the scientific community in Europe. There is no record of James Macleod discussing this aspect of publishing the results of their experiments with either of the researchers in his department.

Throughout the insulin story, as far as Banting's contribution goes, what stands out is his desperate desire to find the extract as soon as possible and to use it as a treatment for diabetes in the desperately ill patients. Even the mention of the possibility of winning the Nobel Prize did not appear to have had any important or lasting influence on the young Canadian.

This emphasis in Banting's motivation of bringing insulin to the suffering distinguishes him from most, if not all, other researchers involved in the pursuit of an effective pancreatic extract before and during the time when the experiments were being carried out in Toronto.

According to Alfred Nobel's 1895 will, each of the five separate prizes, including The Nobel Prize for Physiology or Medicine specified that the prize/s are awarded "to those who, during the preceding year, have conferred the greatest benefit to humankind".

Therefore, if one were to interpret the rule literally, that alone would call into question the claims of some of the scientists involved in the pursuit of insulin. It must be remembered that in the year following it's trial on the patient in Toronto General Hospital in January 1922, hundreds of patients especially in Canada had benefited from the use of insulin which within weeks had transformed the health of scores of patients and, in many cases, had saved their lives.

Delays due to further testing would have resulted in the death of many of these patients who received insulin in the first few months, following its demonstrable benefit in Toronto in January 1922.

In fact, further trials were being undertaken in England, where insulin had been supplied by the Toronto team but was withheld from patients until the English authorities were certain of the safety of the newly developed treatment. Bliss in his book recorded the case of the daughter of a prominent churchman in London who lost her life during that period when the English physicians and scientists waited for the results of the trials being carried out in England at the time when it was already being used on patients in the United States.

Early figures following the use of insulin showed that the life expectancy of young people with diabetes, had risen from an average of five years to 26 years, a truly remarkable early result of using insulin.

It is no exaggeration to say that insulin had removed the "miasma of despair" which had haunted the patients affected by diabetes as well as their families before the discovery of insulin and the demonstration of its dramatic effectiveness in the treatment of the feared condition.

32

AFTER THE REJOICING, THE REALITIES

The lifesaving and life changing effects of insulin were understandably, recognised and celebrated throughout the world. Also applauded were the efforts of the team from Toronto who had made the discovery, and started providing the insulin extracts as quickly as they were made, to patients in Canada mostly at the army hospital in Toronto where Banting was working. The lives of some of the men and women who were rescued from almost certain early death have been written about in newspapers and books. Some have been described in this work.

However, the joy of the rescue was tempered by the realities of the price paid. The needles caused pain and local infections including abscesses. Insulin itself caused low blood sugar reactions, "hypos". Gradual improvements in the quality of insulin addressed many of these difficulties. Further improvements continued and culminated in the form of insulin which is used today. That is part of the story of modern insulin.

Even after the discovery of insulin, a diet limited in starches (carbohydrates) remained the cornerstone of treatment of diabetes.

The use of tablets for the treatment of various ailments was well known at the time of the discovery of insulin but early attempts to treat diabetes with tablets had frustrated physicians and pharmacists over the years.

Even before the discovery of insulin, a group of tablets released on European markets as *Phenformin* which was discovered in 1919 to lower blood glucose but was withdrawn when it was discovered that it could cause damage to the liver.

In the 1950s, further refinements of phenformin led to the development of *Metformin* which is still used in the treatment of adults with diabetes. Even today many physicians consider Metformin to be the treatment of choice in adults with diabetes.

Newer tablets have come on the market regularly since the 1950s to the present day.

With the increasing number of adults with Type Two diabetes, the use of tablets occupies a prominent place in the treatment of millions of individuals around the world.

Recently, there has been considerable publicity because one of the newer agents *Semaglutide* (with trade names Ozempic, Wegovy, Rybelsus), was found to lower the body weight of patients suffering from obesity without diabetes. The costs for this were prohibitive for many patients. In some countries the medication was provided through government-subsidised health services. Its availability on the open market led to non-diabetic individuals purchasing the product to lose weight for cosmetic reasons which resulted in a shortage of supplies for patients with diabetes.

Animal insulins remained the mainstay of the treatment of insulin-requiring diabetes till around 1980. Transition to the new forms varied from country to country.

Even though modern insulin, to be described next, was discovered in the laboratory in 1971, its availability to patients had to await mass manufacturing by pharmaceutical firms.

It is generally agreed that without the involvement of the pharmaceutical industry many of the discoveries may not have been made, at least at that particular time.

33

THE MIRACLE OF INSULIN

The effect of insulin being available to treat diabetes cannot be overstated. The literature in medical, as well as lay publications is full of exuberant praise for the life-changing effects insulin. Expressions such as "near resurrection" and "a miracle" were plentiful in the recognition of the breakthrough in Toronto.

The helplessness of doctors, as well as the patients before the discovery of Insulin was reflected in the preface of the first textbook of the treatment of diabetes written in 1916 by Elliott Proctor Joslin of Boston. The title, *The Treatment of Diabetes Mellitus With Observations Upon The Disease Based Upon One Thousand Cases* was clarified in the preface which began with the following sentence:

> "In writing this book, I have tried to record those facts which have proven of service to me in the treatment of diabetes. For the benefit of my patients it has seemed well worthwhile to summarise my work with them during the last 18 years, and I have honestly tried in these pages to let the <u>400 fatal cases tell their useful lessons to the 600 living</u>."
>
> (Underline by the writer).

The author's excitement was based on the effectiveness, albeit at a cost, of treating patients with diabetes with a restricted diet as employed by Dr. F.M Allen of the Rockefeller Institute for Medical Research which, according to Joslin, had "decidedly changed the outlook for this class of patients."

What may understandably shock today's reader would be the fact that out of the first thousand patients 400 had died.

It is difficult for us in the 21ˢᵗ-century, given all the advances in treatment, to truly comprehend the patient's and the doctor's awareness of the helplessness and confusion, and the quiet anticipation of the inevitable outcome in many of the afflicted as described in Joslin's patients.

In terms of cold statistics, it can be stated that before the discovery of insulin the lifespan of most young people including children with diabetes was four to five years – sometimes even less – but following its discovery the use of insulin transformed the outlook to a life expectancy of an individual with that affliction to around 25 years. Thus, within the first few years of its use, the number of patients with diabetes whose lives had been saved by insulin could be counted in millions. Little wonder that the discovery was hailed throughout the world, and words like a "miracle" or "near resurrection", were being used especially by doctors who had experienced and watched the suffering of countless individuals including children as well as their parents in the years before the discovery of insulin.

Remember that diabetes had been wreaking havoc on mankind since the time of the pharaohs.

These facts alone would support the awarding of the Nobel Prize to the discoverers of insulin.

Just as important were the continuing efforts to improve the preparation from the form which was used initially.

The very thought of piercing one's child, with a sharp needle several times a day was a constant heartache for the parents of children with diabetes.

Insulin had to be injected by needles which were attached to syringes. This was the original method until the newer forms of giving insulin, which include insulin "pens", insulin pumps (where the insulin supply is carried in a small device attached to the patient), and jet injectors were developed.

Newer methods being worked on at present, include taking insulin by inhalation or insulin contained in compounds which can be swallowed. Research into these continues with the hope of being able to take insulin without the need to inject it.

The second preoccupation of users and doctors alike was to discover a way to make the effect of insulin last longer so as to reduce the number of injections the patient needed to have every 24 hours.

It took 14 years after the discovery of insulin to accomplish this through the development of Protamine Zinc Insulin (PZI).

The background to the story introduces several individuals who played an important part in the introduction of insulin in Europe. They were also involved in significant improvements in insulin and its use in patients with diabetes.

In 1936, Hans Christian Hagedorn (1888–1971), developed a combination of insulin with protamine, the latter derived from the sperm of fish (trout), which slowed the absorption of the insulin so that the effect lasted between 14 to 24 hours.

Following the discovery of insulin in Toronto, Hagedorn had given up medical practice to concentrate on developing and refining instrument. The Danish physician remained involved in this aspect of the treatment of diabetes to the end of his life.

In 1939, David Aylman Scott in Toronto, found that adding zinc to Hagedorn's preparation made the compound more stable and increased the duration of its effect of lowering blood levels of glucose. Protamine Zinc Insulin (PZI), in some instances, lasted for 48 hours.

The importance of this discovery to the patients who were using insulin in the early years of diabetes is difficult to describe. The parents of children and the nurses and doctors involved in their care could not find enough superlatives to applaud the practical importance of this discovery.

Thus after some 14 years of using insulin in its original form, patients with diabetes, instead of having up to four even six injections every 24 hours were able to have just one or two injections a day.

Elliott Joslin hailed Hagedorn's discovery as the beginning of a new era in the treatment of diabetes. just as he had named the period of the dietary treatment of diabetes based on the teachings of his German mentor as the Naunyn Era, Joslin maintained that the introduction of the insulin preparation introduced by the Scandinavian had heralded the Hagedorn Era.

In the early 1950s, more new preparations of insulin were produced in Denmark by Knud Hallas-Moller, Thorvald and Harald Pederson, and Jürgen Schlichtkrull. Their work resulted in the introduction of Lente insulins.

Together with isophane insulin, also called Neutral Protamine Hagedorn (NPH) these preparations achieved acceptable control of blood sugar levels in patients with diabetes with only one or two injections every 24 hours. These insulin preparations remained the mainstay of the daily treatment of the majority of patients with diabetes throughout the world for the next 60 years until the discovery of modern insulin.

A first-hand account of using insulin in 1923.

One of the few first hand accounts – and the only one I could find – on the use of insulin at the time of its discovery comes from none other than Robert Lawrence himself as quoted in the 13th edition of Joslin's Diabetes Mellitus (editors C.Ronald Kahn and Gordon C.Weir, 1994.)

> *"When I started insulin in early 1923, nearly 24 years ago, it had only begun to come into commercial production in England....*
>
> *About April 1923, wasted, thin, fit for nothing, in a cautious way I began to use insulin... I understood that there was enough for me in my hospital to carry me on for about a month, then the grace of God would have to supply me with a new set-up. But something developed. A girl (a doctor's daughter) in diabetic coma was admitted. To bring her out, she got the insulin on which I had hoped to live the next fortnight. Well, I was in a jam....*

Somebody somehow brought me a bottle of Lilly insulin the next day. I looked at it with suspicion, but I was glad to have that, really – anything with an insulin label on the bottle. By the end of the fortnight, I had complete confidence (in the new insulin), which I have never had any reason to change in the supervening years."

The Enigma of Insulin.

For centuries, insulin had dwelled within the deepest recesses of the offals of animals slaughtered for human consumption. The offal was discarded, and lay on the floor of abattoirs to be swept up as garbage.

The discovery of insulin is the story of the remarkable changes in the fortunes of a humble hormone.

A Sad Footnote. The Story of a 23-year old English Butcher.

William Davies (1831–1921) was an Englishman who had immigrated to Canada at the age of 23 years, and later founded the William Davies Company which packed meat products, mainly pork. At one stage, his business was the largest pork packer in the British Empire and had led to Toronto's nickname "hog town" because of the large number, reaching into the millions, of pigs slaughtered annually by the Toronto company.

It was to the abattoirs of the William Davies Company that Banting and Best used to go, usually on Saturday mornings, to collect the discarded offal which contained sweetbreads (including the pancreas), heart, liver, tongue, and kidney. In the laboratory, they separated the pancreas from the rest of the offal which was fed to the dogs being used for their experiments.

The sad footnote to the insulin story is that William Davies whose company continued to supply the raw product – later imposing a cost on the offal when he realised it's potential for being used medically – did not live to learn of the life-changing effects of insulin made from the discarded animal products in his abattoirs. a few months before the announcement of the discovery of insulin in 1921 by the Toronto researchers, Davies died as a result of injuries sustained when he was butted by an aggressive goat.

34

TEACHERS, MENTORS, EXEMPLARS

"Man is only a reed, the weakest in nature, but he is a thinking reed."

Blaise Pascal (1623–1662). Theologian, mathematician, philosopher and physicist who invented the syringe in 1650.

The word mentor is derived from Greek mythology. A man called Mentor was given the responsibility of teaching, caring for, and overseeing in general, Telemachus, the son of the Greek king Odysseus when the latter went to the Trojan War.

When used as a common noun, the word describes a person with the dual attributes of a capacity for influencing young men and women by providing knowledge through instruction.

In this particular work which is on a medical subject, the history of mentoring may be more apt in the story of a different Greek scholar.

A "mentor", an individual, and the act of "mentoring," are terms which have become popular and come into greater use in the second half of the 1900s. A mentor is an experienced - usually older - person who helps a younger member of a team at work to facilitate his or her progress. "Mentoring" is a common practice in the modern workplace.

Chiron was known for his knowledge of the "medical arts." Asclepius, the Greek god of doctors, had also been instructed by Chiron who had cared for him and had instructed him in "the art of healing."

Chiron was more widely known than Mentor and is credited with guiding the young Achilles who went on to achieve considerable distinction as a warrior who conquered Hector in the Trojan War.

Often forgotten are the many men and women who have guided young physicians and scientists during their studies of different aspects of diabetes ranging from the early years following graduation to later appointments in research Institutions. Many medical graduates – provided they could afford to travel – left the United States to visit prominent medical universities institutions to observe the treatment of patients there as well as to seek the advice and guidance of senior researchers and professors in Europe, especially Germany and France.

With the passage of time and the growth of the larger centres of learning, particularly through universities and medical schools attached to hospitals particularly in the United States and Britain, the senior men and women provided guidance and opportunities for local younger graduates as well.

Most of the men and women in this book were influenced, even inspired, by their teachers who included professors in Europe. Europe, especially Germany and France attracted a steady stream of such medical students and graduates. For example, William Osler had learned much from Rudolf Virchow, the German professor often referred to as "the father of modern pathology" who was also a respected anthropologist, pathologist, prehistorian, writer, and politician. (Ref. *Sir William Osler An Encyclopaedia* p.811).

Two Inspirational Women in the Journey of Diabetes and Insulin.

Alice Hamilton (1869–1970).
The First Woman Admitted to Harvard's Medical Faculty- *but not to the Harvard Club.*

> *The magic of being a man still counts for a great deal in the medical profession.*
> *New York Tribune. April 6, 1919.*

> *"I chose it because as a doctor I could go anywhere*
> *I pleased – to far off lands, or to city slums – and be*
> *quite sure, I could be of use anywhere."*
> *Alice Hamilton on her decision to study Medicine.*

As World War I ended with victory to the Allies, another significant victory was the appointment of a woman on the staff of the Harvard medical faculty.

When the Dean of the Harvard Medical School, David L. Edsall, discussed appointing a woman to a teaching position, the Harvard President Abbott Lawrence Lowell was less than enthusiastic. In the end, he agreed with the proviso that "she is really the best person for it in the country."

The appointment was widely reported.

On March 12, 1919, the New York Times reported that "the first woman to hold a position on the Harvard University Faculty will be Dr. Alice Hamilton of Chicago.

The Boston Globe added its own tuppenny's worth,"the bars are down! Spring millinery will be a feature of Harvard faculty meetings henceforth" it declared.

The New York Tribune commented that Hamilton must have "great talent; otherwise, the overseers would have had no trouble in overlooking her. The magic of being a man still counts for a great deal in the medical profession."

The Board of Overseers announced that Hamilton would be the Assistant Professor of Industrial Medicine. Hamilton was the first woman on the Harvard Faculty. She was 50 years old.

Ironically, the university at that time did not admit women students. Hamilton's appointment came with three stipulations:

1. She could not march in the Commencement procession,
2. She was not allowed to attend the faculty Club, and
3. She was not going to be assigned any tickets to the Harvard football games.

Hamilton had a way with words. For example, when commenting on the toxic work environment for women, she said, "there's too much chivalry outdoors, and too little indoors."

Late in life, at age 88, she said, "for me the satisfaction is that things are better now, and I had some part in it."

Hamilton's advice to Richard Minot which took place during the First World War when Minot was serving as a surgeon in the US Army, was to look carefully into the working conditions of the workers at munitions factory in New Jersey. They were eventually found to be suffering from ailments which could be traced to skin contact with TNT. Minot later credited Hamilton for her guidance which he said taught him the value of careful attention to the social and working conditions of subjects in his research projects.

Hamilton's contributions highlighted by her appointment to the Harvard faculty as recounted here also touched on the wider social issue of sexist attitudes towards employment opportunities for women as existed at that time. This issue was re-visited by Roslyn Yalow in her Nobel Lecture.

Rosalyn Yalow (1921–2011).
"A Smart, But Poor New York City Girl."

"It virtually changed the world…"

Jens F. Rehfeld on the development of radioimmunoassay by Berson and Yalow.

Rosalyn Sussman Yalow was born in a poor Jewish household in the Bronx, New York, in 1921, the year of the discovery of insulin.

At that time the only professions open to women were as secretaries or teachers. Yalow taught herself to type and secured a secretarial position at the Columbia University College of Physicians and Surgeons. She had hoped that this would be one way to gain entry into a tertiary institution because what she really wanted to do was to study science because when she was in seventh grade at school, her chemistry teacher had aroused her interest in science. Then she found out that the graduate school would not admit a woman.

Eventually, a biochemist hired her on condition that she studied shorthand - typing.

The enlistment of men to serve in the Second World War in 1939, left many places vacant in universities and therefore positions were offered to women so that the institutions could remain open. Yalow went to the University of Illinois, where she was the only woman in a class of 400, and the first since 1917.

In 1943, Yalow married a fellow student, Aaron, the son of a rabbi. They had two children.

In 1945, though only 24 years old, she had earned a PhD in Nuclear Physics.

In 1947 Yalow joined the veterans administration hospital in the Bronx to develop a department which concentrated on radio isotopes. She did not have a laboratory, but that did not deter her. Instead, she converted a closet, which had been used by a janitor into her first laboratory.

Yalow's major contribution to science was through her collaboration with a medical graduate called Solomon Berson. Starting in 1950, They worked together for 22 years, the partnership ending when Berson died in 1972.

For the discovery of radioimmunoassay and its application to research she was awarded the Nobel Prize for Physiology and Medicine in 1977. Yalow could not share the award with her senior collaborator because the Nobel Committee stipulates that the award cannot be given posthumously.

The development of this technique by Yalow and Solomon Berson in 1960 revolutionised the research into various physiologic and biochemical phenomena. Berson, a medical graduate with no research experience was, according to Yalow, "the most brilliant man I have ever met."

Radioimmunoassay made it possible for researchers, for the very first time, to measure extremely small quantities of different elements in the blood. Since many biological substances, including hormones, are present in the blood in such minute – and hitherto immeasurable – quantities, this new technique enabled scientists to overcome this particular difficulty.

The method was first used in the measurement of and research into the body's handling of injected insulin in patients who had diabetes. The reason for the choice of insulin was that by comparison with other hormones, supplies of insulin in purified form were more easily available.

However, there was also a personal reason for Yalow's interest. Her husband had insulin dependent diabetes.

A year later, radioimmunoassay was used for accurately measuring glucagon, a hormone which counteracts the blood sugar-lowering effect of insulin.

Yalow shunned feminist organisations throughout her life but was a firm believer in advocating a pathway for women in science. She did not subscribe to the popular notion of "balancing career with home life" and was able whenever possible, to incorporate her domestic obligations and duties with her work commitments. Yalow had married Aaron, a Rabbi's son in 1943, and had faithfully kept a kosher home without ever questioning the traditional domestic roles of women including those of motherhood. They had two children.

It is said that she would run home to prepare meals for her two children, Ben and Elanna, and her husband, then return to continue her work in the laboratory.

In her acceptance speech at the Nobel awards, Yalow said, "the world cannot afford the loss of the talents of half its people if we are to solve the many problems which beset us."

35

ORPHANED BY A STRAY BULLET

The Many Journeys of Rachmiel Levine (1910–1998).

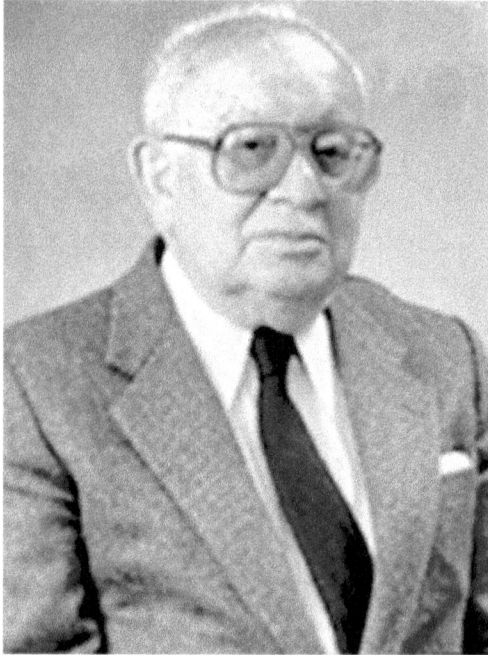

Rachmiel Levine "Father of Modern Diabetes Research."

That mentoring casts its influence beyond teaching is dramatically illustrated in the life of the much admired Rachmiel Levine.

Levine was born in the time of the Austro-Hungarian empire in Czernowich which is now called Chernevtsky in modern day Ukraine.

To call his childhood tumultuous would be an understatement. His mother died in 1914 when Levine was four years old. His father survived World War I but died just after it ended, killed by a stray bullet during an anti-Jewish riot.

Levine was brought to Canada by his grandparents. He went to McGill University from where he graduated with honours in medicine in 1936.

Most of his work was done in the United States, starting with an internship and residency training at the Michael Reese Hospital in Chicago where he worked with Samuel Soskin.

From 1942 to 1960 Levine was the director of the Department of Metabolism and Chairman of the Department of Medicine and director of medical education at Michael Reese Hospital. Later he relocated to New York Medical College where he was the chairman of the Department of Medicine from 1960 to 1971.

Levine's book "Carbohydrate Metabolism" published in 1946 became a stepping stone for researchers working on diabetes.

His description of the role of insulin in glucose metabolism led to his title "Father of Modern Diabetes Research."

Levine's Role in the Modern Insulin Story.

Levine's role in another area of diabetes research may also describe him as a father of *modern* insulin development.

Although much of his work was done at the Michael Reese Hospital in Chicago, Illinois where he had completed his internship and residency training between 1936 and 1938 and then had served as Director of the Department of Metabolism and Chairman of the Department of Medicine and Director of Medical Education between 1942–1960, he had relocated to New York Medical College where he was Chair of the Department of Medicine from 1960 to 1971.

Levine moved to California in 1971 to serve as Executive Medical Director at City of Hope Medical Centre. He served in that capacity for eight years to the end of 1991.

In the early 1970s, when Levine was engaged in projects aimed at developing the diabetes program in the not-for-profit institution, the City of Hope Hospital, Robert Swanson the financier, was working with his team of scientists to develop recombinant insulin. This was a complicated process involving firstly, the development of the recombinant product which was unique in itself, followed by the tortuous process of getting a commercially viable product on the market.

Levine's role in the early stages of the development of modern insulin is detailed in a publication from the Arthur Riggs Diabetes and Metabolism Research Institute in 2022, as well as an article in the Journal of Biological Chemistry (2021, 297 (5) by Kenneth T. Farabaugh).

In 1978, Levine encouraged Keiichi Itakura and Art Riggs from the research division of City of Hope to joined Herb Boyer's team in the early stages of development of human insulin. Although this is mentioned infrequently, Riggs had first heard of Herb Boyer's research on genetic engineering when he had gone to a lecture given by Boyer.

Arguably a more important aspect of Levine's contribution was getting the new insulin to the patient. Remember that Levine was also a medical graduate. He was aware of the need to use a reputable pharmaceutical company to market the revolutionary product. His long experience with medical products had given him an insight into the complicated negotiations which he realised needed to be carried out with a reputable pharmaceutical firm.

Levine was familiar with the long-established Lilly Company and was on friendly terms with its medical director, JHA Clowse. Clowse for his part had known of Levine's research background on insulin during the latter's contributions in earlier studies when Levine was based in Chicago. Levine's reputation in the research community paved the way for Lilly's participation in getting the new insulin to the standard required for getting it into the market, and therefore to patients with diabetes.

This collaboration between Genentech, the research team of Boyer, together with the City of Hope duo Riggs and Itakura was in no small measure due to Levine's encouragement and "people skills" which brought about a collaboration between Boyer's and Swanson's company Genentech and the Lilly Company to bring human insulin to the individuals whose lives depend on the hormone. This is described in the second part of this book.

Thus Levine, the teacher and mentor was an amazing amalgam of a brilliant original thinker in research as well as a friendly "elder statesman" who inspired young men and women to strive for excellence in their research as well as their care of the sick. He also possessed the gift of diplomacy and persuasion in dealing with bureaucracy.

But above all, Rachmiel Levine was blessed with a generosity of spirit which served to bring the best out of people.

Levine retired from the City of Hope at the end of 1991 but continued his involvement with the scientific community throughout his life.

During the 60 years he had devoted to diabetes research and practice, Levine had also served as a mentor and advisor to countless younger colleagues.

His credo was

"a good research scientist needs to have endless curiosity and enormous amounts of patience, since answers in the field of research, come slowly and most painfully."

A Personal Note.

As part of the worldwide celebration of the 50th anniversary of the discovery of insulin, by the Toronto team, Dr. Levine visited Sydney Australia in 1971. It was shortly after my wife and I had returned to Sydney after completing my fellowship in Diabetes and Internal Medicine at the Joslin Clinic in Boston.

One of my colleagues during my time in Boston was Suresh Mehtalia, an accomplished specialist in the treatment of Diabetes, originally from Mumbai, India. Suresh had worked with Levine before coming to Boston. He had told me of the high regard in which the scientist-clinician was held and how popular he was with the younger members of the staff.

During Levine's visit to Sydney, the late Dr. James Isbister, then a senior physician at the Royal North Shore Hospital (in Sydney) hosted a dinner at his home in honour of the distinguished visitor. One of the younger physicians at the dinner happened to comment on the examinations he had recently passed for admission to the Royal Australasian College of Physicians as "a wretched exam".

Levine was quick to react.

"Why do you call it a wretched exam ?" he asked.

Having been told of the distinguished visitor's formidable reputation, the aspiring young physician was too confused to answer.

Levine continued, "exams make you study and learn subjects that you wouldn't otherwise visit in your reading."

Nothing more was said.

Levine died in Boston in 1998 at age of 88.

An Inspiration for Two Nobel Laureates.

Marvin Siperstein (1925–1997).

Here we meet one of the most accomplished scholars of the modern era whose experience and observations in several fields of study on different aspects of diabetes were to play a major part in the evolution of this subject for several decades to come.

An outstanding example of this was the work and influence of Marvin D. Siperstein, a highly respected authority on diabetes and specifically on the metabolism of cholesterol.

Not only did Siperstein train, but, as is a mark of distinction in talented teachers and exemplars he also inspired younger men who came under his influence. This included two of his protégés, Michael Brown and Joseph Goldstein, who went on to win the Nobel Prize for their work on cholesterol. In an interview recorded in the online archives of California, Joseph Goldstein, who later rose to become the Chairman of the Department of Molecular Genetics at the University of Texas Southwestern recalled that "Dr Siperstein first aroused my interest in cholesterol, which has become a lifelong passion." He said that he had found Siperstein's lectures on cholesterol, diabetes, and metabolic disease "among the most stimulating and thought-provoking that I had ever heard."

Marvin Siperstein was a Professor of Internal Medicine and a respected and renowned researcher in diabetes and cholesterol metabolism. The 1985 Nobel Laureates for Medicine and Physiology were Michael Brown and Joseph Goldstein. It was Siperstein's earlier work on the metabolism of cholesterol in the human body which had been further developed by the two Nobel Laureates. They never forgot to acknowledge Siperstein's contribution to their work.

A stickler for correct methodology in scientific investigation, he fearlessly pursued any practice or dogma in scientific investigation, especially if it was being used in patient care. The best known example of this was seen in 1977 when Siperstein together with five colleagues, challenged diabetes researchers and clinicians to provide objective evidence that blood glucose levels of patients with diabetes could be controlled without endangering, those who suffered from the condition, and which would decrease complications of diabetes, especially in those who suffer from diabetes of long duration, as was the case in many, if not most of the so-called Type One diabetes sufferers, who were generally younger than the Type Two patients whose diabetes usually starts in middle age.

Improved technology, which led to the development of ways of self monitoring of blood glucose by patients with diabetes themselves, P paved the way for one of the most important and publicised experiments on patients with diabetes in recent years. It was called the Diabetes Control and Complications Trial (D C C T).

When the results of this trial proved that strict control of the blood sugar level reduced the level of complications, Siperstein's challenge which had played a central role in bringing about the trial, was acknowledged by American Diabetes Association, the leading American body of physicians involved in the treatment of patients with diabetes.

Siperstein had worked firstly in the Southwestern Medical School from 1955 to 1963 when he left to join University of California San Francisco Medical School where he remained till his death in 1997 at the age of 72 years.

The very model of the complete man Siperstein, in addition to his contribution to medical research and teaching medical students, was also devoted to his family and took a keen interest in his home. During one of my visits to his home, he was proud to show me his vegetable garden. A lifelong pursuit of physical fitness accounted for his lithe, compact, physique.

My personal association with Marvin began when I met him after presenting a paper at the International Diabetes Federation's triennial congress in Sydney in 1988. Working with Larry Vogelness, the Chief Veterinary Surgeon of Taronga Park Zoo of Sydney, we had discovered the first example of spontaneous, insulin-requiring diabetes in a chimpanzee. Marvin and I kept in touch after that.

I recall meeting up with Marvin during one of my visits to the University of San Francisco and asking him about the half-marathon which had been run in the city shortly before my trip. I had noticed a news item mentioning the annual event in San Francisco. The journalist had written that the race included running across the Golden Gate Bridge.

When Marvin pulled up in his European model car (a Saab) in front of the hotel where I was staying I noticed that he was in running shoes and athletic wear. When I asked him if he was interested in jogging and what he thought of middle - distance running such as the recent half marathon, Siperstein's response was short, almost sharp.

"That's only 13 miles," he said.

I had not known of his interest in keeping fit through regular running. Nor that he had run a full marathon (26 miles), in Boston in 1976.

There was much more to Marvin Siperstein than his exceptional capabilities in medical research and his inspirational teaching of medical students and graduates. But, as is the case with many such individuals, he never talked about himself.

Marvin Siperstein's son, Alan followed him in the medical profession and currently holds the Chair of Endocrine Surgery Department at the Cleveland Clinic.

Marvin and his wife Eleanor had that special gift of making people feel special, as they made us feel whenever my wife and I visited them at their home in San Francisco.

36

WILLIAM OSLER'S GIFT
TO DIABETES

Osler's role in the insulin story did not escape the attention of his biographers. Both Harvey Cushing in his Pulitzer Prize winning two-volume edition of *The Life of Sir William Osler* which was originally published in 1925, and Michael Bliss in his *William Osler, A Life In Medicine* written more than half a century later in 1999, describe the Canadian physician's uncanny instinct in predicting that medical research would be halted only temporarily by the First World War. As described in this work, Frederick Banting had embarked on his quest for insulin upon returning from his war service in 1919.

Bliss speculated that had Osler lived for three more years "he would have hailed the conquest of myxoedema by thyroid extract…. and the possibility of diabetes being similarly defeated through endocrine research".

Osler would have been transported into ecstasy at the announcement in 1922 of the isolation of the internal secretion of the pancreas and it's almost-miraculous effect in bringing starved, dying children back to life and health. He would have been especially thrilled that the near resurrection happened in Canada, at Toronto General Hospital and the University of Toronto. And he might even have claimed paternity because the clinician who started the Toronto research and shared the Nobel Prize for the discovery of insulin was Fred Banting, son of the William Banting who was baptised in Bond Head by Osler's father, Featherstone Osler on the same day in 1849 that he (Featherstone Osler) christened his own son William. Osler would probably have made jokes about how magically medicated that holy water must have been.

(In 1923 Lady Osler invited Banting to stay at 13 Norham Gardens. Banting was thrilled to have slept Osler's bed.")

Osler made several contributions to the studies of, and developments in, diabetes.

William Osler (1849–1919), had died before insulin was discovered in 1921. Therefore, his comments should be remembered in the context of diabetes still being a condition of unknown cause. Indeed neither the exact source of the factor or factors responsible for causing diabetes, nor the nature of the substance or the hormone at fault had been identified.

At best, there was a suspicion that there was perhaps a substance within the pancreas responsible for controlling the level of glucose (sugar) in the blood.

One may justifiably consider some of William Osler's pronouncements on the subject as *prophecy*, and other suggestions as the result of an unusually penetrating insight – *perspicacity*.

As for his contributions to the insulin story, it may be argued that the most important one was to approach, and then appoint John Jacob Abel (1857–1958) the first full Professorship of Pharmacology at Johns Hopkins in 1893.

In 1925 Abel succeeded in isolating for the very first time, crystals of insulin. The usually taciturn researcher could barely control his excitement, describing the glistening crystals as "one of the most beautiful sights of my life."

Osler's Prophecy.

Harvey Cushing, described by the late Michael Bliss, as "a giant of American medicine, and without doubt, the greatest figure in the history of brain surgery" was a colleague and friend of William Osler. The two had been colleagues at Johns Hopkins before Osler had accepted the invitation to a Professorship at Oxford University in England.

In the second volume of his Pulitzer Prize–winning book *The Life of Sir William Osler* Harvey Cushing revealed that Osler had kept up with the research on diabetes even before the discovery of insulin.

He described Osler's visit to Toronto in mid-1909 to see his relatives when the physicians of Ontario invited him to speak at their annual meeting which was held on June 3rd, 1909.

Osler spoke on "The Treatment of Disease."

This lecture is mentioned because it contains two important statements made by Osler which showed the depth of his thinking on evolving concepts of medicine generally, as well as on medical progress through laboratory research.

Firstly he pointed out how the conception of disease had changed since ancient times and that the new concept had "radically altered" the practice of medicine. Choosing tuberculosis as an example Osler declared that the profession had substituted "the open air and dietetic treatment for the nauseous mixtures with which our patients were formerly drenched."

Secondly, he made a statement on the pancreas which was called a "prophecy" by Harvey Cushing.

Osler stated that "as our knowledge of the pancreatic function and carbohydrate metabolism becomes more accurate we shall probably be able to place the treatment of diabetes on a sure foundation."

The same biography of Osler contains an example of the much admired Canadian physician's way with words. Speaking of the anatomy of the gland where insulin is made Osler, when teaching his students used unforgettable phraseology. speaking of the pancreas, he referred to "the area of abdominal romance, where the head of the pancreas lies folded in the arms of the duodenum."

Neither Osler nor indeed any of the physicians of Ontario could have known that in that very city the "sure foundation" of the treatment of diabetes was to be discovered 12 years later in 1921 by another of Osler's countrymen namely, Frederick Grant Banting. As mentioned above, Frederick Banting's father had been baptised by Osler's father on the same day as William Osler himself.

In recognition of Osler's interest in medical history, The Osler Club of London was founded in 1928. It is housed in the premises of the Royal College of Physicians in London. The Club's stated aim is to encourage an interest in the history of medicine. It is a Gentlemen's club with a membership which includes the elite of the medical establishment. It meets regularly and hosts an annual Osler oration.

The American Osler Society is possibly the most active of the Osler societies with a membership (including students) of around 250. In 2020, the Osler Society issued *Sir William Osler An Encyclopaedia,* edited by Charles S. Bryan. The 900 page tome features numerous essays by men and women many of whom knew Osler. My treasured copy of the book was acquired through generosity of my friend, Professor Milton Roxanas, a member of the board of curators of the Osler Library in McGill University.

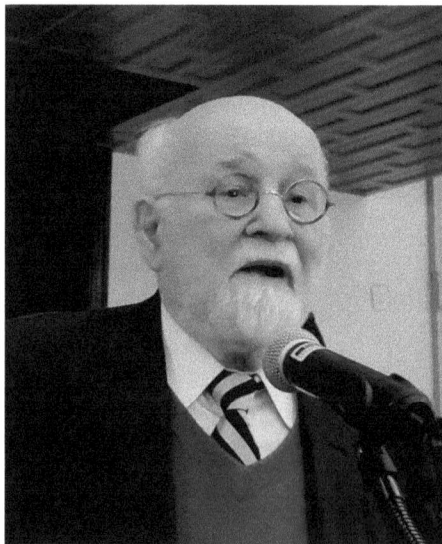

Professor Milton Roxanas.

Sir Edmund Boyd Osler (1845–1924), a Philanthropist Who Helped in the Discovery of Insulin.

Edmund Osler's role in insulin has been seldom described. The only one of the five Osler brothers not to go to university, he chose instead to enter the banking industry. Starting as a bank clerk while still in his teens, he next moved into stockbroking and insurance, but returned to banking in his later years by becoming a shareholder and later, in 1901, a Director of the Dominion Bank.

The discovery of insulin by Banting and his colleagues in Toronto in 1921, the space in the laboratory had to be extended for large-scale production of the hormone to be used to treat the large number of patients with diabetes.

A $500 donation for building the laboratory was given dmund Boyd Osler in 1914. He was at that time on the Board of Governors of the University of Toronto. His donation was used to convert the Museum of Hygiene in the basement of the medical building into three rooms: a general laboratory, a room for washing and sterilising glassware, and a small laboratory for bacteriological examinations. Initially established to produce diphtheria antitoxin its facilities were expanded to increase its output and range of products.

Frederick Banting had used these facilities for part of his experimental work which culminated in the discovery of insulin.

The director of these laboratories, the remarkable John "Jerry" Fitzgerald (1882–1940) was a behind-the-scenes helper and mentor of Frederick Banting.

Edmund Osler retired from politics in 1917, but continued his philanthropic activities to the end of his life. He died in 1924 at age of 78 years.

The Reverend Featherstone Lake Osler (1805–1895) and the coincidence of his baptism of Frederick Banting's father on the same day as baptising, his son William has been mentioned above.

Featherstone Lake Osler, the father of the two other men in this story, was born into an English ship-owning family.

In 1831 Featherstone Lake Osler, was invited to serve on HMS Beagle as the science officer on Charles Darwin's historic voyage to the Galapagos Islands, but could not accept the offer as his father was dying.

He was ordained in 1837 and moved to Canada shortly afterwards. He had a 20 year tenure in Canada.

All his children were born in Canada.

The youngest son William became, at least in the medical world, the most famous of the Oslers.

William Osler is widely regarded as the Father of Modern Medicine.

William Osler's role in the insulin story was through the appointment of John Abel as the foundation professor of pharmacology at the Johns Hopkins Hospital when Osler was the Professor of Medicine.

Abel isolated insulin crystals as recounted in this book. Secondly, his recognition of Elliott Joslin's potential in the early years of the latter's medical practice by including him in the first group of the young physicians when starting the Osler Club, led to unique contributions by the Boston physician to the knowledge of diabetes and its treatment including the use of insulin from the time of its discovery as well as his guidance provided to the Toronto team of Banting and Best. Charles Best remained a friend and admirer of the Boston physician till the end of Joslin's life.

One of William Osler's First Assistants Joseph H. Pratt devoted his life to the study of diabetes. Pratt was prominent in the discussions and controversies at the time of the discovery of insulin by Banting.

37

RUSSELL HENRY CHITTENDEN
(1856 – 1943)

Mentor of Elliott Proctor Joslin.

In the story of diabetes in North America, one of the first such physicians who later specialised in the treatment of diabetes was Elliott Joslin of Boston.

Although Joslin claimed that he had wanted to be a doctor ever since an attack of measles during his childhood his memoir written by the Harvard University librarian Anna Holt described the influence of Chittenden "one of his teachers at Yale", who according to Holt, remained a life-long friend, helper and admirer of Joslin. Russell Chittenden's influence was a reason for Joslin choosing to study medicine. Holt wrote that the Yale professor remained an influence on the ambitious Bostonian even after the latter had finished his college studies.

Referred to by some as "Yale's most distinguished scientist," Chittenden was the leading American authority on what at that time was a new branch of science called "physiology".

Chittenden's own mentor was Willhelm Kuhne (1837–1900), a highly respected scientist, with a faultless academic pedigree. He had studied under Claude Bernard in Paris, and in the laboratory of Rudolph Virchow, "the father of modern pathology." Kuhne had carried out detailed studies on the chemistry of digestion. The charismatic German had been deeply impressed by the quiet 22-year-old Chittenden (even though the American could not speak a word of German) and remained his lifelong confidante, the relationship ending only with Kuhne's death in 1900.

In 1874, Chittenden had introduced a new course which he called Physiological Chemistry. He had designed the curriculum especially for students in their senior year at Yale. It is said that the course proved so popular that "students literally flocked to (Chittenden's) new laboratory."

In a comprehensive essay on Chittenden published by the National Academy of Science the writer said that "Chittenden is credited with influencing a generation of distinguished scholars at Yale and other institutions to do laboratory research work as part of their medical training."

38

BERNHARD NAUNYN
(1839–1925)

This German physician professor was referred to by Elliott Joslin of Boston as the Nestor of diabetes. Nestor, a character from Homer's classic, *The Odyssey* was known for his wisdom and his powers of persuasion which some attributed to his long-winded dissertations, which sometimes led some members of the audience to agree to follow his advice in order to stop him talking!

Naunyn was the son of a wealthy Berlin burgomaster (a German term for a high-ranking city official, like a mayor, or in some cases, the head of a city-state).

He graduated from the University of Berlin with a degree in medicine and started as an assistant to the distinguished pathologist Friedrich von Frerichs (1819–1885) who is remembered for writing the first German textbook on Brights Disease, a chronic ailment which affects the kidneys.

It was during his time with Frerichs, that Naunyn became interested in the pathology of the liver, pancreas and other organs which were to lead to his later interest in and studies on diabetes.

He went on to head the medical clinics in Konigsberg from 1872 to 1888 before moving to Strasbourg where he remained till 1904.

In 1898, Naunyn published an important monograph with the title *Der Diabetes Melitus (sic)*.

From the point of view of diabetes and this book, the most distinguished of Naunyn's students who later served as his assistant, was Oskar Minkowski. The brilliant investigator known for his surgical dexterity who demonstrated that the cause of diabetes lay in the digestive organ pancreas, was also widely regarded as one of the most gifted surgeons of his time.

However, as will be seen later in this account, Minkowski was not able to pinpoint the exact part of the gland wherein lay the cause of diabetes,.

Another of Naunyn's students was Otto Loewi (1873–1961), who won the Nobel Prize in Physiology or Medicine in 1936 for his work on nerve transmission.

Naunyn was one of a group of German physicians who advanced German medicine from an 18th century discipline which held that the study of medicine was part of the discipline of natural philosophy, as was widely believed in the 18th and 19th centuries. The concept of medicine as a science had to be founded upon results of experiments in the laboratory. Furthermore, the validity of the results of experiments was accepted only if repeating the experiment yielded the same result.

Naunyn had been influenced by the Cantani system of treating diabetes with a strict low carbohydrate diet before the discovery of insulin. If patients did not adhere strictly to this principle Cantani is said to have locked them in their rooms for months at a time to keep them away from sugar.

When attending a German medical conference the American diabetes specialist, Frederick Allen, who was a contemporary of Elliott Joslin, called Naunyn "a champion of strict, carbohydrate-free diet."

Even then this was still "a voice in the wilderness." Most of the speakers at the Congress, including several German physicians, were opposed the practice of strict dietary restriction as part of the treatment of diabetes.

In the English-speaking world, Naunyn's method was given prominence mainly by the Boston diabetes specialist Elliott Joslin who had visited Naunyn in Strasburg 1896 at the end of his medical course at Harvard University. The German professor had also emphasised the importance of vigorous treatment of even the milder cases of diabetes because of his conviction that this approach delayed, even perhaps prevented the worsening of diabetes.

When his mother, Sarah Proctor Joslin developed diabetes in 1899 at the age of 60, Joslin travelled from Boston to Strasbourg for Naunyn to examine her and advise on her treatment. Accounts of her diabetes are to be found in the diabetic manuals written by Elliott Joslin as well as in his memoir by the Harvard University's librarian Anna Holt (*Elliot Proctor Joslin, A Memoir, 1869–1962 by Anna C.Holt* published privately in 1869 to mark the centenary of Joslin's birth. They describe Joslin's mother keeping strictly to the prescribed diet, which Joslin insisted was the reason for her living a productive life for another 14 years. She died at the age of 74.

Joslin, an avid letter – writer kept in touch with Naunyn throughout the latter's life.

Joslin did not waiver in his belief in strict carbohydrate restriction as the basis of treating diabetes in the years before the discovery of insulin. Some contemporaries and younger diabetes specialists in later years vigorously opposed the strict approach, but the Bostonian never wavered.

It is now part of the history of controversies in Medicine, that many years later, the results of a multi-centre trial referred to as the Diabetes Control and Complications Trial (DCCT) confirmed that strict control of blood sugar did achieve the results as believed by Naunyn, and practised by men like Joslin and Allen.

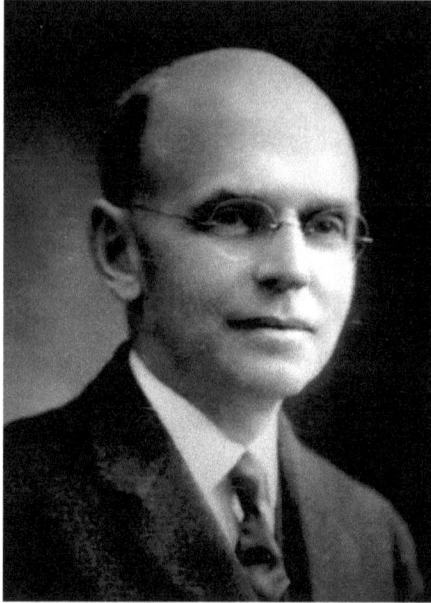

Elliott Proctor Joslin of Boston.

Joslin followed Naunyn's dietary advice throughout his long life which he devoted to the treatment of patients with diabetes. Joslin mentored generations of specialists in diabetes through the fellowships awarded to medical graduates not only of American but foreign medical schools.

He also kept in contact with Naunyn as indicated in a handwritten letter from the latter. I also have a photograph of a handwritten letter to Joslin from Minkowski with information on Naunyn's death.

Naunyn had started a scientific publication, called *Archives of Experimental Pathology and Pharmacology.*

Naunyn's most distinguished associate, and student, was Oscar Minkowski whose story is related in different parts of this account. Minkowski remained with Naunyn till the latter's death.

39

A PHYSICIAN AHEAD OF HIS TIME

Apollinaire Bouchardat (1809–1886).

Regarded by many as the leading diabetologist of the 19th century, Bouchardat's medical education had started as an assistant in his uncle's pharmacy. He went to Paris at age 19 to study medicine, and was nominated as professor of hygiene at the Faculte de Medicine in 1933.

Bouchardat became the chief pharmacist at Hotel Dieu in 1835. It was from his workplace at the hospital, that Bouchardat saw the dispirited, defeated soldiers of the French army, returning from the Franco-Prussian war.* He remembered the emaciated men and women with diabetes who had consulted him during the siege of Paris. He had recognised in them what to him was a silver lining but which he did not divulge to the patients given the sense of despair which had pervaded the city during the siege. Nevertheless, he was astonished that these patients with diabetes had markedly diminished amounts of sugar in their urine. Some produced urine without even a trace of sugar.

Starvation had improved their diabetes.

Bouchardat was one of the first physicians to address specific issues of treatment for diabetes.

He was an early pioneer in advocating *education* as part of the program for the treatment of patients with Type 2 diabetes.

Having seen the effects of *weight loss* as recounted above Bouchardat emphasised the importance of achieving sugar-free urine through weight loss. He was probably the first physician to recognise the importance of this in patients with diabetes, and an issue in the management of the condition which has remained important, perhaps even more so now because of the high incidence of obesity throughout the world especially in the developed nations.

Thirdly, he was the first to include *exercise* in the program of treating patients with diabetes telling them that "one must exercise, preferably three times a day, long enough to get warm, but not tired."

Lastly, and for that time quite revolutionary, was Bouchardat's suggestion that *the patient take responsibility for the treatment and overall management of his condition, rather than simply carrying out the orders of the physician.*

It is said that he never wrote about this in any of the information given to patients in later years, when he publicised reduced food intake and exercise to clear the urine of glucose.

Another piece of advice by this physician, not widely known except in his clinic, was that he allowed his patients to have red wine once their urine was free of sugar but reminded them to reduce, if not stop the intake of "the nectar of the grape" when sugar reappeared in their urine samples.

Bouchardat was also one of the earliest workers in the field to hypothesise that diabetes originated in the pancreas long before Oskar Minkowski's and Josef von Merring's seminal contribution by the dramatic demonstration of diabetes in a previously normal dog after the surgical removal of the animal's pancreas.

In 1875 Bouchardat published one of the earliest textbooks on diabetes with a second edition in 1883 more than a decade before Naunyn's 1898 treatise on the subject.

True to the mission of the institution where he worked, Bouchardat provided medical care to patients who came to Hotel Dieu to the end of his life.

It is said that in his final years this pioneer of diabetes lived in poverty.

Bouchardat died on April 7, 1886. He is buried in the Pere-Lachaise Cemetery in Paris.

I was told by the late Dr Robert F. Bradley, President of the Joslin Clinic in Boston that the institution's founder Dr. Elliott Joslin, whenever he visited Paris, never left without visiting Bouchardat's grave.

It is also interesting that, although Joslin admired the Frenchman and used his method of dietary restriction and exercise, the staunch puritanical New Englander who was a strict teetotaller, never advocated or even tolerated wine in the dietary regime of his patients. He persuaded them to follow a strict diet, and to exercise regularly, often repeating Bouchardat's recommendation, but there is no mention of wine as having any part in Joslin's treatment of his patients, nor in the treatment manuals he wrote for patients, or the textbooks of diabetes he regularly issued for physicians over a period of forty plus years.

*The Franco German War (also called Franco-Prussian War), July 1870 – May 1871, pitted a coalition of German states against France, which ended in the defeat of France thus ending its superior position, "hegemony" in Europe at the same time as leading to a unified Germany.

The chancellor at the time, Otto von Bismarck, a consummate and wily politician had, according to some sources, been the architect of the conflict and had brought it about through secretly altering some of the communication with the French emperor Napoleon the Third which drew the emperor into the war which he had been reluctant to join.

The Story of Nobel Laureate Professor George Richard Minot (1885–1950)

"George Minot's case history illustrates the drama and pathos of the "transition" period between the "under-nutrition" treatment of Dr Frederick Allen and the availability of sufficient insulin.

"Saved by insulin was the expression used to describe the fortunate ones" said Donald M. Barnett in *Elliott P. Joslin, MD: A Centennial Portrait* published by the Joslin Diabetes Centre in 1998.

The importance of this account lies in the effect of diabetes in an individual during the period when Minot's diabetes was discovered because his condition had to be treated without insulin. Although discovered that summer in Toronto, Canada, insulin had not been sufficiently refined in quality nor produced in quantities adequate for the needs of patients outside the immediate vicinity of the Canadian laboratory where the earliest supplies were being produced.

Minot's story touches on several other aspects of diabetes. Through him we meet remarkable individuals who contributed to the understanding of diabetes at that time and continued to do so through their care of patients with the condition. These were practising physicians. Later, progress in medical practice had reached the stage at least in parts of America, that research workers, who had qualified as medical graduates, made further contributions to the understanding and treatment of diabetes. The story of some of these men and women are also presented here.

Minot came from one of the aristocratic Boston families often referred to as Boston Brahmins. His father, James Jackson Minot (1853–1938) was a physician and a professor at Harvard university. He had been one of the teachers of Elliott Joslin, at that time, one was the few physicians in the United States to specialise in the treatment of diabetes.

The young professor had a happy home life having married Marian Weld in 1915.

An important part of this story is the extraordinary effort on the part of his wife who mastered not only the basics of diabetes but also the details of its treatment, especially the diet that needed to be followed. Every account of his life includes descriptions of the contributions made by his wife to her husband's successful handling of the day-to-day challenges faced in the treatment of his condition.

Minot's story is also recounted because of the dramatic circumstances of his rescue from almost certain death by the use of the recently discovered insulin.

Minot had graduated from Harvard Medical School and trained at Massachusetts General Hospital. However his plans were suddenly interrupted in October 1921 when at the age of 36 he was alarmed by days when he started to feel excessively tired, weak and thirsty. He tested his urine for sugar and was alarmed by the strongly positive test.

He knew that he had diabetes.

The very next day Minot went to the highly respected Boston physician Elliott P. Joslin who confirmed that Minot had indeed developed severe diabetes.

The only form of treatment was semi-starvation which offered survival at the cost of profound loss of weight and a crippling loss of energy in most patients. The sight, especially of young men, women, and children, crippled by a lack of energy, and having the appearance of starved individuals broke the hearts of all who saw them. Some commented that the experience reminded them of the photographs of prisoners in concentration camps during wartime.

In October 1921, when the 36-year-old was found to have diabetes, insulin was only just beginning to enter the conversation. Even then, as described in this account, the discussion was largely based on word-of-mouth stories of what was supposed to be happening "up there in Toronto" as Banting's research was referred to by the Boston diabetes specialist, Elliott Joslin.

The symptoms of hypoglycaemia are usually overcome with a small amount of sugar in the form of a sweet drink or a candy which most patients carry for precisely this purpose.

For Minot, the frequent bouts of hypoglycaemia may also be put down to the emphasis on keeping the blood sugar as close to normal as possible being stressed by his physician Elliot Joslin. Also, Minot being a physician, understood the importance of that advice and attempted to minimise high blood sugar levels.

From the viewpoint of the story of diabetes Minot's illness serves as a memorable account of the fate of patients with diabetes before and after insulin was made available for treating the condition after its discovery by Frederick Banting and his colleagues in Toronto in 1921.

Joslin, already recognised as an expert on diabetes, had enjoyed a privileged association and friendship with the young researchers Frederick Banting and his student helper, Charles Best. Thus he was able to obtain supplies of insulin before it became available to the general public in the United States (in 1924). Minot was given insulin in early January 1923. At first the cautious physician only gave 1 or 2 units at a time until buoyed by its prompt effect not only on the blood sugar levels, but more importantly, on the increased energy it gave the patient, Joslin eventually increased to dose to 18 units before breakfast, and 14 units at bedtime. For the first time since the beginning of his diabetes Minot *felt better* with more energy and gradual increase in strength and weight. Within twelve months Minot's wife, as quoted by Barnett said,"this is the first winter, since marriage, that he has not lost 7 - 14 days from his illness."

Minot returned to his research activities, including the directorship of the prestigious Thorndike research laboratory in 1928.

In the August 14, 1926 publication of the Journal of the American Medical Association I found an article with the title "Treatment of Pernicious Anaemia by a Special Diet."

The authors, George Minot and William P. Murphy announced the discovery of an effective treatment for the hitherto fatal Pernicious Anaemia.

Minot's research efforts in the field of haematology are best remembered for this discovery of an effective treatment of Pernicious Anaemia with liver extracts.

Minot was rewarded for the discovery with a share of the Nobel Prize in 1934. The co- recipients for their work on the same project were George Hoyt Whipple and William P. Murphy.

Before the discovery of this treatment, pernicious anaemia had caused the death of thousands of patients around the world.

William Castle, a renowned haematologist said that insulin not only saved the lives of the millions of men, women and children who had suffered from the hitherto fatal condition but by saving Minot, the cure for Pernicious Anaemia, also until then fatal, probably saved even greater numbers of human beings around the world.

Insulin does not solve all the problems of diabetes, and this is well illustrated in Richard Minot's case history. His conscientiousness in using insulin to keep his sugar level as close to normal as possible often led to attacks of hypoglycaemia which in Minot's case caused abrupt personality changes, most commonly causing him to become extremely angry. His wife's unwavering support throughout his life is documented and commented on by Joslin and several of his junior physicians, including Barnett.

Elliott Joslin placed the photograph of Minot as the frontispiece in the 10th edition of the diabetic manual for patients with diabetes written in 1959.

Minot died on February 25, 1950 aged 65. He had lived a successful life, some would say a brilliant life, and had managed his diabetes for nearly 30 years during the early years of the use of daily insulin injections. In 1956 Rackemann wrote a biography of Minot with the title *The Inquisitive Physician.*

A Modern Day Professor Speaks of His Diabetes.

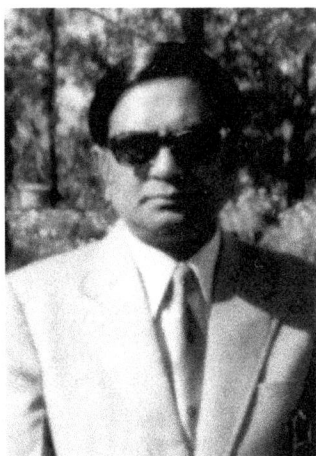

Professor Munichoodappa (1938–)

Professor Munichoodappa, Muni to me, has been a friend since our time together in Boston, USA in1969 when we were awarded fellowships for further studies in endocrinology, especially diabetes at the Joslin Diabetes Centre, known at that time as the Joslin Clinic. After completing his fellowship, Professor Munichoodappa returned to India. He has lived and worked in Bengaluru (previously called Bangalore), throughout his professional life.

Some years ago, Muni told me that he had suffered from diabetes from the age of 40, and had treated it with diet. He was generous with the details of his condition but surprised me when he casually remarked that in his opinion, nerve damage (neuropathy) in diabetes, at least in some instances maybe hereditary. In spite of my own interest in that particular complication of diabetes, I had not heard that it was familial. I didn't ask him whether he had told me that to catch me off guard, at which over the years, he has succeeded more than once ! However, I had to admit that the particular association he spoke of was new to me.

When I embarked on this project, I asked, not without hesitation, if I could include his observations in this account. I respect the many individuals who are reluctant to reveal personal details to an unknown audience. I received an answer within 24 hours saying, "Of course you can. Here are the details.

"I am 85 years old now and have had diabetes since 1980 from the age 40 years."

I am on a strict diet even though on festival days and on birthdays I have small quantities of some sweets. I exercise daily, walking about 1 km and am active throughout the day in my practice, I inject myself with a mixture of long acting and short acting insulin every day. For burning in my feet, I have used *pregabalin* which has helped.

My laboratory tests, including cholesterol, haemoglobin A1c (a measure of the level of high blood glucose in the blood) and tests on my kidney, and my heart (electrocardiogram) are normal.

Family History.

I come from a family of three sisters and I am one of four brothers. All of us have diabetes.

My mother had diabetes.

My maternal grandfather also had diabetes. He was an active man in his village in Tamil Nadu.

My grandfather had developed diabetes at the age of 80+ My children are all free from diabetes. My son (also a specialist in diabetes) plays golf 3 to 4 times a week.

My brothers' children and some of my sisters' children have also developed diabetes.

The origin I think is my maternal grandfather. He refused to take medications but remained on a diet and was physically active. He died at the age of 90 when I was in Boston at the Joslin clinic."

Damage to nerves in the lower limbs, specially the feet and the lower half of the legs often referred to as diabetic sensory neuropathy is a well known complication of diabetes.

However, as yet there is no firm evidence that it affects other members of the family across generations as it clearly has in Professor Munichoodappa's family.

An Interesting Coincidence.

The Annals of Internal Medicine is a medical journal, which publishes scientific articles on medical subjects. The articles are written by practising physicians and research workers.

The journal dates it's beginnings from the early years of the last century.

The Annals of Internal Medicine was established in 1927 by the American College of Physicians , an organisation formed in 1915 and modelled on the Royal College of Physicians of London, which had been founded in 1518 by a Royal Charter granted by the well-known (and much maligned) King Henry the Eighth.

On 1 October 1970, *The Annals of Internal Medicine* carried an article with the following title:

Diabetes Mellitus and Pernicious Anaemia. C. Munichoodappa MD; George P. Kozak. MD, FACP.

I'm sure the fortuitous connection with the discoverer of the treatment of Pernicious Anaemia and his own observations on the subject some fifty years later would not have escaped Professor Munichoodappa.

40

A BEND IN THE RIVER

Rivers have intrigued many well known writers ranging from Leo Tolstoy (1828–1920) to V.S. Naipaul (1932–2018). Tolstoy saw in a river, elements it had in common with human beings: clear and bubbling in some aspects, deep and inscrutable in others. The Indian novelist, Naipaul in his novel *A Bend in the River* described in memorable prose the profound changes which occurred in the lives of the villagers who lived on a river bank beyond the bend compared with those who lived in the upper reaches of the waterway. A similar profound change which occurred in the journey of diabetes is described next.

The Early Years of Insulin Treatment. A Brief Retrospective.

Even in the early 1970s in Australia, where diabetic patients were treated in the outpatient clinics of the larger hospitals, deep abscesses were seen at the injection sites in the buttocks of children. The injections of insulin in the early days were also painful. Before disposable needles were manufactured, the needles often had to be sharpened manually.

A particularly troublesome aspect of the early insulin preparations was the short duration of action. Blood sugar could only be lowered for around four hours, sometimes less. This meant that injections had to be given three or four times during the day and often, also during the night.

The needles had to be sterilised and the syringes, which in the early years were made of glass, had to be cleaned and sterilised before use.

So although insulin saved lives, the early methods of using it were a challenge not only for the suffering but also for those who had to care for them.

The use of the original insulin preparations often referred to as soluble, or quick acting insulin were the only preparations available from the time of the discovery in 1921 until 1936 when the first long acting preparation achieved through the addition of protamine and zinc to insulin resulting in PZI (Protamine Zinc Insulin) was produced largely through the efforts of Hans Christian Hagedorn in Denmark.

The refinements in the duration of different preparations of insulin led to medium acting preparations, which permitted the control of diabetes to be achieved with one or two injections during the day.

Having spent my entire professional life, using the old insulin and seeing the results firsthand as well as knowing of its life-saving and life-giving effect on literally hundreds and thousands of patients around the world, I realise that in spite of the shortcomings as described above, insulin was a vast improvement on what it had replaced.

A simpler way of looking at the dramatic improvement achieved by insulin in the treatment of diabetes was that insulin changed the previously fatal condition to an illness which although not curable, could be controlled and allowed patients to live longer lives.

Insulin allowed children to grow into adulthood, pursue careers, marry and have families and, like other members of the community, attend school and university. Some of the accomplishments of such men and women are part of this account.

Events Preceding the Development of Modern Insulin.

Although the discovery of insulin heralded relief and joy because of its lifesaving effect on thousands of patients with diabetes, the actual nature of insulin itself remained a mystery.

Mukherjee, referred to insulin as "the Gabor" of hormones perhaps because when she had been seen in an American film in the 1920s, the actress Greta Garbo had been described as "the most mysterious of Hollywood stars." In 1981, more than 50 years later, an article in Variety magazine said that the screen goddess "still remains the most elusive, mysterious and speculated about film personality on the planet…"

That insulin lay undiscovered within the human body for literally thousands of years, also reminds one of the fable of Cinderella which dates back to the writings of a Greek scholar as early as 23 CE.

The modern version started in 1812 in Germany when the Grimm brothers published their version in *Grimm's Fairytales*.

Worldwide publicity followed the release in 1950 of the Disney film *Cinderella* based on a French version of the story in which Cinderella is trapped within a step-family from which she is rescued by a prince.

As in the case of Cinderella, the transformation of insulin into a life-saving and life transforming 'elixir' following its discovery within the innards of pigs and cattle has continued to fascinate students of history and science. (Just what the reaction of Fred Banting, the decorated soldier would be to being thought of as a prince, I will leave to the reader, but I suspect it would be entirely acceptable to his many admirers in Canada who remain loyal to him to the present day).

From the lonely occupant of the discarded innards of offal on the floor of the abattoirs of the Davies Company in Toronto to the pinnacle of biotechnological research, the celebrated molecule's journey has captured the interest of chemists, molecular biochemists and scholars from then to the present day.

It is truly a story of a remarkable transformation.

Little wonder then that those of a religious persuasion, like the Boston physician Elliott Joslin, invoked biblical analogies when describing insulin's discovery in the "pancreatic juice".

The discovery also caused great excitement in the research community because scientists now had a protein to investigate.

The mass production of insulin made it easy and inexpensive to obtain supplies of the hormone from pharmaceutical firms for researchers to investigate various aspects of its structure.

Insulin quickly became the "go-to hormone" for the modern day scientists and compared with what followed especially with the advent of modern techniques and technology, the earlier attempts including those used by Banting and Best in Toronto were almost rudimentary.

The excitement and anticipation caused by the discovery of insulin was not restricted only to those who were suffering from diabetes and their families and carers. The revelation of the hitherto suspected, but stubbornly elusive, secret dweller within an equally frustrating hiding place in the pancreas opened the floodgates of inquiry within the medical and scientific communities around the world.

Insulin was the word on everyone's lips. The worldwide news coverage of the success of the previously unheard-of Toronto workers was echoed in the local newspapers of countries all around the globe. After all, diabetes was not restricted to any racial or geographic group. By the time of the discovery of insulin in 1921, the ancient ailment had moved out of the history of the early civilisations to afflict the children and adults of virtually every continent and island around the globe.

The discovery of insulin was a scientific breakthrough on several fronts:

Insulin was the first protein the nature of which was revealed through the the prize winning – and backbreaking – efforts of the Cambridge scientist Frederick Sanger who discovered a method to determine the order of the arrangement, *sequence*, of the individual proteins (amino acids) in the hormone.

Insulin was the first hormone upon which x-ray crystallography was used by Dorothy Hodgkin to demonstrate its three-dimensional structure. (She had returned to work on insulin after researching penicillin because of its usefulness during World War Two).

Insulin was the first hormone measured by radioimmunoassay, a Nobel Prize-winning scientific method developed by Solomon Berson and Roslyn Yalow.

Finally, modern insulin was the first mammalian DNA which was cloned by David Goeddel through recombinant technology pioneered by Paul Berg.

In short, insulin had opened the floodgates of Research.

Modern insulin was also unique in that it had been introduced on the stock market with spectacular results and had led to the launching of the biotechnology industry. By contrast, the patent for insulin discovered in Toronto had been sold to Toronto university for one dollar.

In retrospect it is clear that the discovery of insulin in Toronto in 1921 had provided a springboard for intensive research by scientists in several branches of chemistry and biochemistry which culminated in the successful development of the modern model of the hormone which is now used by millions of patients throughout the world to treat their diabetes.

As sometimes happens with a bend in the direction of a river, a profound change in the journeys of diabetes and insulin has taken place over a period of the past 30 to 40 years. The change saw the previously less common Type 2 diabetes, affecting a larger number of patients thus overtaking Type1.

Furthermore, those individuals who developed Type 2 diabetes were adults and not children as had been the case with Type 1 diabetes.

According to the National Institute of Health (NIH) the total number of patients with diabetes in the world was in the order of 462 million in 2017. Of these, Type Two diabetes made up 90 to 95% of the total number.

The critical difference from the point of view of treatment between Type Two over Type One diabetes is that is that *Type Two diabetes does not need insulin as part of its treatment.*

Type Two diabetes is generally controlled with a calorie-restricted diet, reduction in body weight, increased physical exercise and the use of medications which in most instances are tablets to be taken by mouth and not by injection as was, and remains, the case with insulin.

The reason for Type 2 diabetes overtaking Type 1 is generally attributed to changes in "lifestyle" which, through a combination of increased food intake and diminished physical activity, has led to a marked increase in the incidence of obesity.

Nor is diabetes a disease of the wealthy. It now poses a challenge for virtually every country in the world including the Third World nations.

A common factor underlying this explosion is *obesity*.

The ready availability of "fast food" has been identified as an important underlying cause. Strategies, including exercise, improved nutrition and lower caloric intake supplemented by different medications are being advocated in an attempt to stop this worrying trend.

Increased resources especially in countries where healthcare is funded by the government as it is in the United States of America have enabled researchers to identify previously unknown underlying factors responsible for the change.

The parts played by different organs, including the liver, muscle and fatty tissue as well as the islets of Langerhans are among the areas being studied with the aim of finding drugs which would assist in the treatment of an increasing number of patients with Type Two diabetes.

The subject of tablets in the treatment of diabetes which began in the late 1960s is now an important part of the story of diabetes.

Several classes of drugs acting through different pathways in the body are now part of the treatment used in the management of the millions of patients with Type Two Diabetes around the world.

At least eight mechanisms in the human body have been identified as playing a significant role in causing Type 2 diabetes and have been labelled "the ominous octet." (Ref. Chaudhury A. et al).

At least six or seven different classes of medications are now available for the treatment of Type 2 diabetes, a far cry from the early days of the use of sulphonylureas in the first half of the 1900s.

The large number of agents now available for the treatment of diabetes, has been the result of a greater understanding of the way insulin works in (and on) different parts of the body and the many ways glucose is used by different organs including muscle, liver, brain and kidneys.

Inspite of its history of being in and out of favour over the years, in terms of usage around the world, Metformin, arguably remains the most frequently used medication for Type Two Diabetes.

Insulin however, remains the mainstay of treatment of Type One diabetes. The story of the journey of modern insulin brings us to the next part of this work.

Part Four

Modern Insulin's Limitless Horizons

41

AN EARLY PROMISE

John Jacob Abel (1857–1938).

> *"One of the most beautiful sights of my life."*
> John Jacob Abel, describing insulin crystals in
> December 1925.

The evolution of the original insulin extract through modern advances to the form in which it is used today brings us to the story of modern insulin.

The story of Frederick Sanger, who demystified the actual physical nature (structure) of insulin is, chronologically, the beginning of the scientific scrutiny of this hormone. Next was Dorothy Hodgkin's dogged pursuit over nearly forty years which revealed the structure of insulin. Finally, the team of Solomon Berson and Roslyn Yalow developed radioimmunoassay, a brilliant discovery which opened yet another door to reveal hitherto undiscovered substances which had existed in amounts previously inaccessible because they had been present in minute quantities, or in physically small, often ignored or discarded parts, as had been shown in the early accounts of the search for insulin within the islets of Langerhans.

But first, the story of a man often forgotten in the history of diabetes especially in the pursuit of insulin. It is the story of John Jacob Abel.

Shortly, after the discovery of insulin in Toronto in 1921 the influential Arthur Amos Noyes (1866–1936), a former Professor of Chemistry and Director of the Research Laboratory of Physical Chemistry at the Massachusetts Institute of Technology, who had later moved to work in California, received a grant from the Carnegie Corporation specifically to provide funding for research on insulin.

Noyes knew the scientist who, he believed, was eminently qualified and suited for this project. His name was John Abel, formerly the foundation Professor of Pharmacology at University of Michigan, before he was persuaded by William Osler to join the medical faculty of Johns Hopkins as its first full Professor of Pharmacology.

John Jacob Abel had studied chemistry and physiology at the University of Michigan. After his graduation in 1883 he had spent nearly seven years in several universities and medical schools in Europe. He had studied under, and been guided by, some of the most distinguished teachers there. In addition to Chemistry, Abel had studied Physiology and Clinical Medicine. An intensive two-year period starting in the winter of 1886 at the University of Strasbourg where Abel studied Internal Medicine under the tutorship of Adolf Kussmaul and later, Friederich von Recklinghausen was a life-changing experience for the young graduate.

The University of Strasbourg, which commanded respect and admiration throughout the scientific world counted amongst its alumni, not only scientists like Louis Pasteur, but also others including Albert Schweitzer, the Nobel Laureate with a triple doctorate (theology, music and medicine).

Abel's time in Europe created lasting friendships and relationships with many of his teachers, especially in Germany. His ancestral connections had been in Rhineland. However his American friends always stressed that his loyalties lay in his American roots saying "he remained staunchly American in sentiment and habit of mind."

Upon receiving Noyes' invitation Abel deferred his answer until he had studied the experiments which had previously been performed on insulin. When he replied the answer was typically short and to the point.

"Will attack insulin. JJ Abel."

His experiments showed that sulphur was an integral part of insulin and, perhaps even more importantly, that insulin was a protein and not a vague hitherto incompletely characterised chemical entity which was thought to exist through being loosely attached to, or "adsorbed" on a protein.

In December 1925, Abel was captivated by a vision, which he said was "one of the most beautiful sites of my life." It was the first sighting of the glistening crystals of insulin on the inside surface of a test tube in his laboratory.

Just as important was Abel's demonstration through a chemical reaction called the Biuret Reaction that insulin was a protein.

To emphasise the crystalline nature of insulin Abel's scientific paper submitted to and published in the Proceedings of The National Academy of Sciences in February 1926, carried the title "Crystalline Insulin."

For reasons which are unclear and still unexplained, Abel's contributions to the understanding of insulin have received little acknowledgement, let alone credit.

Next is the story of the discovery and development of a remarkable new technique which was critical in the investigations of, and advances in, the knowledge of insulin as well as other "chemicals" such as antibiotics and vitamins.

42

THE PROFESSOR AND THE POSTMASTER'S DAUGHTER. A COLONIAL DISPATCH

History records the truth of the title of this piece in that William Henry Bragg was indeed a professor and Gwendoline Todd was the daughter of Charles Todd, a postmaster.

In 1889 William Henry Bragg had married Gwendoline Todd.

However, the contributions of both Bragg and Todd were much more substantial and significant than suggested by their "job descriptions" in the title of this chapter.

Charles Todd (1826–1919).

Charles Todd, whose official title on arrival in Australia was Postmaster General of Australia, was in fact an astronomer as well as an electrical engineer and meteorologist. He was born in London. In 1855, at the invitation of the South Australian Government, Todd was nominated by the Royal Astronomer to travel from England to a remote part of the British Empire, namely, the town of Adelaide in South Australia. Todd was charged with the responsibility of establishing a transcontinental telegraph line.

Todd's contributions to meteorology earned him an honorary M.A from the University of Cambridge and in 1889 he was elected a Fellow of the Royal Society. he was knighted in 1893.

Todd's major contributions included the establishment and maintenance of posts and telegraphs in South Australia until federation. This changed with the establishment of the Commonwealth of Australia which then took over all such services in March 1901.

Todd retired in 1906, having served the South Australian and Commonwealth governments for more than 51 years. He had given most of his adult life to serving Australia and did not return to England.

Sir Charles Todd died in his summer home near Adelaide in 1910.

His name appears in many institutions including the Sir Charles Todd building at the University of South Australia, the Sir Charles Todd Observatory, the annual Charles Todd oration held by the Telecommunications Society of Australia, as well as through the naming of Todd river and it's tributary the Charles River in the Northern Territory.

A waterhole – at times referred to as an oasis – in the bed of the Todd river was named Alice Springs after Todd's wife Alice. Later the name was used to name the town established in that area.

William Henry Bragg (1862–1942).

> *"From religion comes a man's purpose; from science his power to achieve it."*
>
> *William Henry Bragg.*

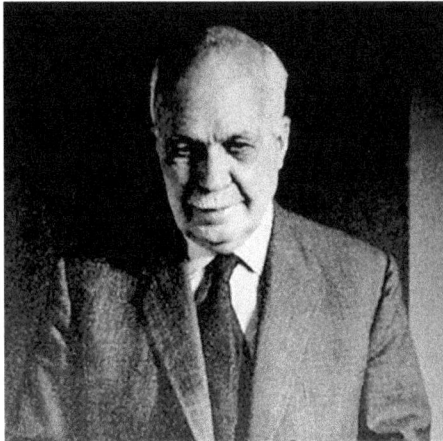

Sir William Henry Bragg (1862–1942).

The many contributions of William Henry Bragg are contained in different parts of this account.

What is often not included in his story was his exceptional gift of the ability to simplify complex scientific information into forms so simple that a child could understand them. One example of Bragg's facility with words which is of particular interest in this account of the exploration of the details of insulin is revealed below.

Being a popular lecturer on scientific subjects, Bragg was invited to give "Christmas lectures" for children. Some of these were published and became "best sellers".

One of these books called *"Concerning The Nature Of Things"* was given to Dorothy Hodgkin on her 16th birthday by her mother. It explained in simple language what crystals were. Hodgkin said that the book helped her to to decide her future which she devoted to working out structures of different proteins through crystallography.

In 1908, William Bragg left Adelaide after 23 years in Australia to take up the Cavendish Chair of Physics at the University of Leeds, which he occupied from 1909 till 1915.

It was during this period that Bragg developed the spectrometer (in1911–1912) which led to the study of crystals, and marked the beginning of the era of crystallography for investigating the inner workings (molecular structure) of drugs such as penicillin as well as hormones including insulin.

The atomic structure of interest in this account is insulin. This was pursued, and eventually revealed due to the assiduous efforts of a remarkable woman who devoted her life to working with crystals. The story of Dorothy Hodgkin is told after the account on crystallography.

43

THE NEW SCIENCE OF CRYSTALLOGRAPHY

I asked the Great Sage, "How can I solve the secret of life?" He replied: "The secret of life lies in the structure of proteins, and there is only one way of solving it, and that is by x-ray crystallography."

Max Perutz, Nobel Laureate.

A concise description of crystallography is as follows: crystallography is a tool through which the precise structure of a crystal can be determined. It works on the principle of crystals causing a beam of x-rays to scatter (diffract) in many specific directions. Then, by using a mathematical formula, it is possible to construct a three-dimensional model or diagram of the atomic structure of the crystal.

The United Nations declared 2014 to be "The International Year of Crystallography." A review article in the scientific journal FEBS - Federation of European Biochemical Societies - published in April of that year included the historical perspective and the achievements of crystallographers which had led to major advances through revealing the details of the structures of various biological substances including insulin.

Particularly useful was a table, which listed the Nobel prizes awarded to various researchers and scientists who had used crystallography to reveal hitherto unknown features of various chemical substances including insulin, antibiotics such as penicillin, and vitamins which had in turn led to further developments including their uses in treating a wide variety of illnesses.

Starting with Wilhelm Conrad Roentgen who was awarded the first Nobel Prize for Physics in 1901 for the discovery of x-rays, the list includes William Henry Bragg and William Lawrence Bragg, the father and son who were awarded the Nobel Prize for Physics in 1915 for the pioneering work on crystallography.

In 1964, Dorothy Hodgkin won the Nobel Prize for chemistry, for her work on several biochemical substances including vitamin B, 12. Her work on insulin came later, towards the end of her illustrious career as described in this work.

The list includes a veritable Who's Who of molecular chemistry, such as Linus Pauling (1901–1994) for Chemistry in 1954, followed by Crick and Watson in 1962 for their discovery of the molecular structure of DNA. All in all the list of Nobel laureates numbers in excess of 40 scientists who had employed crystallography to conduct their research.

Crystallography eventually unlocked the many mysteries of insulin which had defied all earlier attempts at understanding it's inner make–up.

A Father and Son Team in the Insulin Story.

William Henry Bragg (1862–1942).
William Lawrence Bragg (1890–1971).

> *"Nobel Prize for Physics, 1915, awarded to you and your father."*
> Aurivillius, Secretary, Academy of Science."
> The Nobel Foundation.

X-ray crystallography allows the scientist to see the structure of molecules by beaming x-rays through a crystal onto a photographic plate which records a scatter pattern. The process is repeated with a variety of selected orientations. Then mathematical calculations are used to relate the spots on the plate to the relative arrangements of the atoms.

After their discovery by Wilhelm Roentgen in 1895, X-rays became the most prominent method of research in crystallography which was to become a tool for investigating minute structures in nature. Before its development scientists could not overcome the difficulty of understanding the minute scale of action and properties of atoms. Nor could they understand how such minute structures existed in space. For this groundbreaking discovery Roentgen was awarded the first Nobel Prize for Physics in 1901.

When Max von Laue (1879–1960) showed that x-rays are diffracted in crystals and formed characteristic patterns on photographic film, he proved in a single experiment that x-rays are wave-like in nature, and that crystals have a lattice-like structure.

For this work, he was awarded the Nobel Prize for Physics in 1914.

It was not clear whether the structure of crystals and wave-lengths of x-rays had any influence on the diffraction pattern.

That connection was shown by the father and son collaboration between William Henry Bragg and his son, William Lawrence Bragg. The father had designed the first ionisation spectrometer in 1912 which provided an instrument for determination of crystal structures. The son, William Lawrence Bragg, in 1912 demonstrated the Bragg law of x-ray diffraction which permits determination of crystal structure. The wide ranging practical applications of their discovery were clear to the scientific fraternity, and both the Braggs were awarded the Nobel Prize for Physics in 1915. They remain the only father-son recipients of the prestigious award. William Lawrence Bragg was 25 years old at the time. He is still the youngest winner of the Nobel Prize for Physics.

The critical element of the Braggs' breakthrough was that crystals are made of regular, repeating patterns of atoms, like oranges packed in a box. Instead of tackling the complexity of each individual atom's contribution to the x-ray diffraction pattern, the Braggs, through a mathematical formula, (the Bragg Hypothesis) could predict the diffraction pattern from the reflections from each successive plane of atoms within the crystals.

The Braggs used the device to analyse several substances and small molecules using mathematical relationships between the x-ray diffraction pattern, and the arrangement of atoms in a crystal which produced the pattern.

The Braggs' findings in turn led to the new and revolutionary science of x-ray crystallography which for the first time in the history of molecular chemistry made possible the determination of molecular structures of crystals in a compound. Researchers could then actually study crystalline atoms which caused a beam of x-ray to deflect in many directions.

It was from a photograph, the famous Photo 51, which demonstrated the double helix structure of DNA obtained through the use of crystallography by Dr. Rosalind Franklin at King's College, Cambridge that her fellow researchers Francis Crick and James Watson were able to discover the three-dimensional double helix in 1953.

The controversy over Franklin being ignored for the Nobel Prize given to Crick and Watson continues to the present day.

In June 1913, William Lawrence Bragg submitted a paper, "notes", to the Royal Society, describing the reflection aspect of the diffraction of light when directed on crystals. He had found that the planes which contained large number of atoms, provided more prominent diffraction spots. This observation suggested a way of working out the atomic arrangement inside a molecule from these spots. Lawrence Bragg, through this method had found a way to determine the make-up (structure) of crystals.

In 1913, by using a diffractometer the Braggs started determining the structure of different crystals.

From then on x-ray diffraction became the basic method for determining the three-dimensional structure of synthetic and natural compounds.

It was this method which was used to determine the structure of insulin. The work was carried out by Dorothy Crowfoot Hodgkin (1910–1994), the only British woman to win the Nobel Prize.

Modern Insulin. The Early Years.

Of particular relevance to the development of modern insulin were the experiments carried out by three distinguished scientists.

Frederick Sanger. (1918–2013).

In 1958, Cambridge scientist Frederick Sanger, won the Nobel Prize for chemistry for working out the exact order of the arrangement (the sequence) of the basic units of protein, the amino acids, which make up insulin. Perhaps even more important was the discovery by Sanger of a *method* to read the sequence of amino acids. The method, now computerised, is still in use.

Frederick Sanger's painstaking research which clarified the structure of insulin was first brought to the notice of the research community when they were published in 1951 and 1952, and for which he was awarded the Nobel Prize in Chemistry in 1958.

Dorothy Hodgkin.

In 1964, Dorothy Hodgkin became the first and only British woman to win the Nobel Prize for Chemistry for working out the structure of Vitamin B12 which cures Pernicious Anaemia. The condition was fatal before the discovery of its treatment with Vitamin B 12.

In 1969 Hodgkin, 34 years after she had first started on the project, returned to the task of elucidating the structure of the insulin molecule.

Rosalyn Yalow.

In 1977, Rosalyn Yalow won the Nobel Prize in Medicine/Physiology for developing the revolutionary method called radio- immunoassay (R.A.I.) which she and Solomon Berson, her research partner and guide, used for measuring minute amounts of insulin in the blood. The amounts were so small that before the discovery of this method they were undetectable. The method for using this method was published by the two researchers in 1960.

The stories of these three scientists and their contributions are important in the early stages of the development of modern insulin.

44

A NIGHTWALKER IN CAMBRIDGE

Frederick Sanger (1918–2013).

The pride of place in the early critical developments in understanding the actual make-up or structure of insulin is unquestionably held by Frederick Sanger.

Sanger, an Englishman was the son of a general practitioner who had been a medical missionary in China and was of Quaker persuasion. Quakers are Christian but eschew religious conventions and church hierarchy. Sanger himself never formally accepted Quakerism as his religion, but followed many of its principles such as a lifelong opposition to war.

This more than another oft- quoted incident in Sanger's life was the reason for the scientist's opposition to war. At the age of 17 and prior to going to college Sanger had gone to a German school in southern Germany on an exchange program. He was surprised that the school, Schule Schloss Salem began each day with readings from Hitler's *Mein Kampf* followed by the Nazi salute.

In 1936 Sanger started at St John's College, Cambridge enrolling in a course on Natural Sciences. His father had attended the same college to study medicine.

Unhappy with his choices – he found physics and mathematics challenging – Sanger switched from physics to physiology in his second year and went on to biochemistry at which he excelled, graduating with first class honours.

The death of his parents – his father at 60 and his mother at 58 – during the Sanger's first two years of his course at Cambridge gave the young student a substantial inheritance as his mother had come from a wealthy family which had interests in the cotton industry.

Fortunately for science in general and diabetes in particular, the unexpected financial windfall enabled Sanger to change his mind from going on to teaching which he had chosen having realised that he couldn't remain at university because of his limited financial resources. He returned to Cambridge to continue his studies in biochemistry.

Sanger's Research on Insulin.

In 1943 Sanger started working in Cambridge with a protein chemist called Albert Chibnall.

Chibnall, whose interest was in amino acids, had worked on the amino acid composition of bovine insulin. He gave his young protege the assignment of identifying the composition of insulin.

Sanger used insulin obtained from the pancreas of pigs just as the Toronto researchers had done. Whether or not he was aware of John Jacob Abel's work in 1926, when the Johns Hopkins pharmacologist had shown that insulin was a protein which existed as crystals is unclear.

The work which brought Sanger to the notice of the scientific world was carried out in a small, damp, poorly ventilated hut-like laboratory situated in the Fens of Cambridge.

The early history of Cambridge includes a description of this area as a marshy region of nearly 4000 km². The fens are still prone to flooding as they were in earlier years.

The early dwellers believed that the marshy areas were home to ghosts called the "lantern men" who were feared as evil spirits which condemned their victims to death by drowning them in the reed beds of the Fens. Whether it was Sanger's familiarity with the values espoused by Quakers or his own fearless and confident personality is unclear. Suffice it to say that he walked through that area in the dead of night probably so preoccupied with his scientific project as to be hardly aware of the superstitions regarding the lantern men.

In those years people also visited the fens to worship in the monasteries which had been built there over the years.

In the modern era, the only prominent cathedral in the area is the Ely Cathedral, which boasts of its association with the incomparable orator, writer and poet, John Donne who preached there in the 1600s. Donne (1572–1631) was the Dean of Saint Paul's Cathedral.

Sanger never measured the hours he spent in the laboratory. Often he worked through the night, returning home in the early hours for a short nap, before returning to the laboratory.

Not surprisingly, at the end of his career, Sanger graciously acknowledged the support of his wife who had cared for him during the long years of research he had carried out in this dark and damp laboratory.

How many long years, well may you ask?

I'll give you a clue.

There was not a single murmur of complaint or questioning when Sanger was the sole recipient of the Nobel Prize for Chemistry in 1958. Even today, the Englishman's dedication to his task as manifested in his capacity for the sustained effort needed to reach his goal draws gasps of incredulity followed by unstinting praise.

Such determination and capacity for sustained effort over such a long period was unlikely to be affected by stories of the Lantern men or any other evil spirits.

The details of insulin as revealed by Sanger's experiments may be summarised as follows.

Every protein is made up of a number of individual units called amino acid. For a particular protein the amino acids are arranged in a specific order called the *sequence.*

Unlike many other products needed for scientific work, insulin supplies following the discovery of the hormone in Toronto more than 20 years earlier were easily obtained. In Britain, one of the prominent retailers was the well-established pharmacy chain of Boots Chemists. Sanger, like his supervisor Chibnall, worked with bovine insulin.

Sanger's experiments demonstrated that insulin consisted of 2 chains, called the A and B chains which were made up of amino acids in a particular order – sequence –rather like beads in a necklace.

Before Sanger, all attempts at working out the actual nature of insulin had failed.

What Sanger did was dissolve insulin in a solution, then using a particular solvent, he broke off each amino acid and identified it. He would then repeat the process – remove the next amino acid and identify that. The Sanger method for carrying out this part of the experiment is still in use albeit with some modifications made through modern technology.

In this way, by 1955 Sanger had worked out the exact arrangement – the sequence – of each amino acid in the two chains, A and B, of insulin. This, for the first time, revealed that the actual make-up of insulin: the A chain consisting of 21 amino acids and the B chain which is made up of 30 amino acids.

The time-consuming and energy-sapping exercise had taken the dogged Englishmen ten years of "hard labour"in the damp and poorly equipped laboratory near the fens in Cambridge.

Sanger's landmark discovery was recognised by the Nobel Committee which awarded Sanger the first of his two Nobel prizes in 1958. The 1958 award was for his landmark research on insulin.

Sanger's Second Life. Meeting an earlier Nobel Laureate.

Even though Sanger won the Nobel Prize for this work, the accomplished biochemist, being self-effacing by nature, did not regard these experiments as particularly impressive when compared with his next project.

In 1962, Sanger moved to a different laboratory in Cambridge. It was Cavendish Laboratory in the Medical Research Council (MRC) building. Equipped with modern facilities, the new workplace equipped with the latest state-of-the -art facilities was a far cry from the Spartan quarters where he had laboured night and day for ten years to unravel insulin.

The Second Bragg in the Insulin Story.

The role of the father and son team of William Henry Bragg and William Lawrence Bragg in the development of crystallography has been related earlier. At that time Lawrence Bragg was only in his 20s.

Given the auspicious start to his career it is not surprising that Lawrence Bragg rose to be the Director of the Cavendish Laboratory in Cambridge. The Cavendish counted in its ranks the likes of Francis Crick and James Watson as well as Rosalind Franklin and the South African, Sydney Brenner. No prizes for guessing what their focus was - DNA.

Lawrence Bragg was there in February 1953 when the double helix structure of DNA was revealed by the team which included James D. Watson, Francis Crick and Maurice Wilkins, winners of the Nobel Prize for Physiology or Medicine in 1962. Lawrence Bragg had left Cambridge in 1954 but is said to have remained in touch with what was going on at the Cavendish Laboratory.

The role of the famous photograph 51 taken by Rosalind Franklin which was used to discover the double helix has remained a controversial, even contentious subject of many scientific articles as well as discussions in scientific circles. Franklin being left out when it came to awarding the Nobel Prize remains a subject of speculation and difference of opinion.

In the mid 1960s, Sanger started working on nucleic acids. These are large molecules which are present in all known forms of life. DNA mentioned above and RNA (ribonucleic acid) are the two main classes of nucleic acids.

For determining the sequence of a component (bases) in nucleic acids, Sanger won his second Nobel Prize in 1980 which was shared with Paul Berg and Walter Gilbert.

I mention this firstly because Sanger was, and remains, one of the few scientists to win the Nobel Prize twice. He is the only scientist in history to win the Nobel Prize in Chemistry twice.

Paul Berg and Walter Gilbert will feature prominently in insulin's journey at a later stage after further revelations of its "shape and size" revealed through studies carried out by Dorothy Hodgkin.

Sanger remained at the MRC to the end of his life. He retired in 1983, at the age of 65. He was offered a knighthood which he refused, saying, "I don't want to be different."

In1986 he was awarded the Order of Merit which he accepted. It is an honour which can only have 24 living members.

In 1992, The Wellcome Trust and the Medical Research Council (MRC) established the Sanger Centre, which is now called the Sanger Institute. He agreed to open it himself on the 4th of October 1993.

The Sanger Institute is considered one of the leading establishments to have played an important role in the sequencing of the human genome.

The much admired scientist died in his sleep in 2013 at the age of 95. One of the many individuals who had admired Sanger's accomplishments and came to pay their respects to the scientist at his funeral was the father of recombinant technology, Paul Berg who eulogised the Englishman who in spite of his many accomplishments remained humble to the very end of his life.

Composing his own obituary, Sanger wrote that he was "academically not brilliant."

45

A BEAUTIFUL YOUNG WOMAN BECOMES A FAMOUS SCIENTIST

Dorothy Crowfoot Hodgkin (1910–1994).

"I was captured for life by chemistry and by crystals."
Dorothy Hodgkin.

Crystallography enabled Dorothy Hodgkin to reveal the structure of insulin. The connection with William Henry Bragg has been mentioned above.

Although born in England, as a child Dorothy had spent a good deal of time in colonial North Africa where her father was in the Colonial Civil Service. She often played in a creek behind their home in Khartoum and was fascinated by small rocks and stones she found there. She often recounted the story of finding a shiny black rock in a stream which ran in their backyard in Khartoum and asking a family friend, who was a soil chemist, if she could analyse that. The chemist gave her a surveyor's box of reagents and a few minerals to encourage her in her pursuit. Neither he, nor the inquisitive little girl, could have known that the small gesture of kindness was the beginning of a lifelong pursuit of crystals by Dorothy Hodgkin.

At the age of 10, Dorothy and her classmates made solutions containing copper sulphate, which in time produced crystals. So the seeds of this particular aspect of chemistry had been sown during childhood.

William Bragg's book had helped her through explaining how crystals were examined with the use of x-ray. The book was to set her course in life. Referring to these incidents in her early years, she later declared that she had been "captured for life by chemistry and by crystals."

At 18, Hodgkin had enrolled in Oxford University to study chemistry so as to pursue her interest in crystallography. Her supervisor J.D. Bernal had photographed the first x-ray of a protein crystal in 1934. Bernal had been one of William Henry Bragg's students.

Dorothy Hodgkin, who went on to become a highly respected Oxford University tutor – one of her pupils was the late Margaret Thatcher, Prime Minister of England from 1975 to 1990 – was indeed remarkable for many reasons.

The FEB Journal review mentioned above attributed her "truly monumental" contributions to her dual mastery of chemistry and crystallography.

Her contributions to the understanding of insulin came after she had won the Nobel Prize for Chemistry in 1964.

The review also noted that "insulin became her lifelong interest, crowned eventually after almost 35 years of effort by solving the structure of this important protein hormone."

The article spoke of Hodgkin remaining involved in her studies on insulin until the end of her active, scientific career, and also pointed out that she had, in 1988, published probably the longest paper in the history of protein crystallography, which had taken up the whole issue of *Philosophical Transactions of the Royal Society of London, Series B.*

Although the shape of insulin crystals had been described earlier after their discovery by John Jacob Abel who, unlike Hodgkin, had received little recognition let alone praise for his work, the actual configuration of insulin had frustrated all previous attempts.

Hodgkin used crystallography to solve the riddle. Her method of positioning the crystals for her studies is still used today.

The English scientist Frederick Sanger, also a Nobel Laureate for his work on insulin, had influenced Hodgkin through his discovery of the exact order (*sequence*) of amino acids which are the building blocks of insulin.

Hodgkin's interest in insulin can be traced to a meeting with Robert Robinson (later Sir Robert Robinson) in 1934 when Robinson, who had earlier held the position of the Foundation Professor of Chemistry at the University of Sydney in Australia, had offered Hodgkin a small sample of crystalline insulin.

Sir Robert Robinson (1886–1975), a chemist and a Nobel Laureate was a titan of chemistry who was the President of the Royal Society between 1945 and 1950 when women were first elected fellows. Dorothy Hodgkin was elected in 1947.

At that time she knew little about insulin but even a brief reading on the biochemistry of the hormone amazed her because of the number of processes which were influenced by it.

Initially daunted by the size of the insulin molecule, Hodgkin changed direction, and leaving insulin, switched to work on penicillin and later, Vitamin B 12 because both of these were smaller molecules but also because working on penicillin was important as part of the war effort during the Second World War (19 39–1945).

The size of the challenge which Hodgkin had found intimidating several years earlier becomes a little easier to grasp when it is revealed that the number of atoms in a single molecule of insulin is 788.

The difference in the size of the molecules is more dramatically shown by the number of basic units, atoms, in a single molecule of each of these three subjects of Hodgkin's studies. Penicillin has 17 atoms and Vitamin B 12 is made up of 181 atoms. It had taken Hodgkin four years to work out the structure of penicillin. The bigger molecule of vitamin B 12 took eight years of assiduous laboratory work to demonstrate its three-dimensional structure. This particular vitamin will feature in another part of this book.

The Nobel Prize for Chemistry awarded to Hodgkin in 1964 was for her work on Vitamin B 12, which at the time was the largest crystal structure to be revealed by crystallography.

In 1969, 35 years after her earlier studies on insulin, Hodgkin returned to complete the project and demonstrated the structure of insulin. Her discovery played an important role in the mass production of insulin. This was of critical and practical importance to millions of patients with diabetes, their daily requirements of the hormone being dependent on its availability, which in turn required a reliable supply of the hormone.

Hodgkin, who had a strong humanitarian, some say missionary, streak in her personality considered her work on insulin to be the most important, probably because of the number of patients with diabetes who were helped by the advances resulting from her work on the hormone.

Her pioneering work on insulin was to bear fruit through its mass manufacturing within a decade of her contributions.

A measure of her tenacity and determination is seen in her contributions to the crystallography of the three subjects of her scientific endeavours.

She had started her work on insulin in 1934 when she was 24 years old but deferred it because of the more urgent task of working on penicillin because of its use in World War II. It was the simplest of the three structures on her interest. Penicillin had only 17 atoms, but it still took Hodgkin four years to map its structure. Her work was of critical importance in later developments of the antibiotic. She had worked on the structure of penicillin in 1946.

Next she worked on Vitamin B 12, which contains 181 atoms. This work took eight years to map and ended successfully in 1956.

Vitamin B12 itself has a particular place in the insulin story as will be seen in the accounts of the Nobel Laureate Richard Minot and a modern day diabetologist, Professor Munichoodappa of Bangalore, India.

In 1964, Hodgkin was awarded the Nobel Prize for Chemistry "for her determination by x-ray techniques of the structures of important biochemical substances."

Specifically, her method of positioning the images obtained through crystallography became a model followed by other workers engaged in that branch of research.

There is a story about Hodgkin sitting on the steps of the Royal Society with her friend and mentor J.D.Bernal after she had completed her work on penicillin. Bernal, who was popularly known as "Sage" because of his prodigious knowledge of a wide variety of scientific subjects, predicted that she would win the Nobel Prize for her work on penicillin. Hodgkin said that she would prefer to be elected as a Fellow of the Royal Society.

As it turned out, Bernal was right but so was Hodgkin. She was elected to the Royal Society in 1947 and won the Nobel prize in 1964. She also received the Royal Medal in 1956, and the highly prized Order of Merit in 1965.

The high regard in which two scientists involved in researching insulin were held by the English scientific community is reflected in two of their number namely, Frederick Sanger, and Dorothy Hodgkin receiving the Order of Merit.

The Order of Merit was founded by King Edward VII in 1902. It is considered a very special distinction reserved for British subjects considered to have made exceptional contributions in the areas of arts, learning, literature, and science. The number of living holders of this exclusive distinction is limited to 24.

Dorothy Hodgkin was only the second woman to receive the honour. Florence Nightingale was the first to be so acknowledged in 1907.

In 1968 Hodgkin returned to complete her work on insulin, which contains 788 items. She completed her detailed studies in mapping insulin in 1969.

It had taken her 34 years to conquer its structure.

Hodgkin's work on insulin opened the door to remarkable advances in the treatment of diabetes with the hormone.

The reason for Hodgkin putting off her work on insulin after having started it during the time of the Second World War has generally been attributed to her previous work being put aside in order to work on compounds such as antibiotics which were needed as part of the war effort. All of this is true. However, when I was revising this book and preparing the postscript on oral history, I discovered through Hodgkin herself, when she was talking about this part of her work, revealing that an important reason to defer her work on insulin was that the equipment which was used for crystallography in the earlier period needed to be further developed before she could tackle the large molecule of insulin, and it was the later refinement of the machinery that had allowed her to return to her work on insulin in the 1960s.

Dorothy Hodgkin's work on penicillin saved the lives of countless human beings suffering from a variety of bacterial infections.

Similarly, the work on vitamin B12, also transformed the lives of thousands who suffered from the previously fatal pernicious anaemia.

Once again, she had used x-ray crystallography to demonstrate the structure of Cobalamin commonly referred to as Vitamin B 12.

In 1964 she became the first British woman to be awarded the Nobel Prize in Chemistry because of the work which solved the atomic structure of insulin, penicillin and vitamin B12.

What is less well known is the physical toll her work took on Hodgkin. The long years of work in the laboratory had gradually worsened the painful (rheumatoid) arthritis which affected her hands and had been present since she was in her 20s. It was while she was studying for her PhD in 1934 that she had sought Specialist advice on her pain in the hands which turned out to be due to rheumatoid arthritis. Rest was advised, but ignored by the research scientist.

Towards the end of her life, her hands were markedly deformed which made the use of her fingers almost impossible.

Dorothy Hodgkin's remarkable scientific achievements are better known than her devotion to her children. In spite of suffering constant pain in her hands, when away from her children, she wrote to them every day.

Hodgkin was also active in social issues. She had supported and encouraged the American Nobel Laureate (in Chemistry) Linus Pauling in his opposition to atomic warfare, which resulted in Pauling winning a second Nobel - the Nobel Peace Prize in 1963.

Dorothy Hodgkin died in 1994 at the age of 84. Max Perutz, the Nobel Prize winning crystallographer when speaking of Hodgkin said, "there was magic about her person ... like the spring."

46

RADIOIMMUNOASSAY AND INSULIN

The 1977 Nobel Prize for Physiology or Medicine honoured Roslyn Yalow for "the development of radioimmunoassays of peptide hormones". The hormone which Yalow and Berson had used in their experiments was insulin.

Radioimmunoassay is a method for detecting infinitesimal amounts of a substance, such as insulin, in a given sample of blood or serum. For example, it enables scientists to measure one trillionth of a gram of material from one millilitre of blood. The widespread use of radioimmunoassay is due to this characteristic.

Radioimmunoassay was devised by two scientists, Solomon Berson, a physician and Roslyn Yalow, a physicist.

By 1959, they had perfected their method and had used it to measure the level of insulin in the blood of patients who had diabetes.

Radioimmunoassay provided a huge impetus to research in many fields including medicine and, as described here, specifically in clarifying the way insulin works in normal human beings as well as those who have diabetes.

As noted above insulin was the first hormone studied with the use of radioimmunoassays.

This revolutionary technique revealed several previously unknown facts about insulin as it existed in the human body. One of the important findings was made by the researcher, Donald Steiner, who by the use of radioimmunoassay was able to show that insulin existed in the body of humans as well as animals in an earlier form, a precursor, known as *proinsulin*. The same methodology also showed that there are substances in the intestines of normal human beings which play an important part in the way insulin works. This has come into prominence in 2022 and 2023 through the use of newly developed drugs which act in the gut and influence appetite.

Unfortunately, Yalow's friend and mentor Solomon Berson had died some years earlier, and therefore was not eligible to share the Nobel Prize won by Yalow.

Roslyn Yalow never failed to acknowledge her colleague whenever she spoke of their research.

47

A STAR IN A GALAXY

Paul Berg (1923–2023).

> *I was like a child playing with pebbles on the beach while the vast ocean of truth lay before me.*
>
> Sir Isaac Newton, 1643–1727.

> *"I have been to the mountain top. And I have looked over… and seen the Promised Land."*
>
> Martin Luther King, 1929–1968.

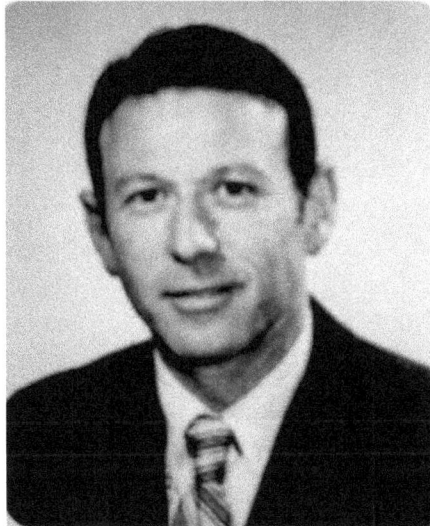

Paul Berg (1926–2023).

Long before Christopher Columbus had crossed uncharted oceans in his ship the *Santa Maria* to discover the New World in 1492, centuries of suffering from diabetes had already been visited upon mankind.

Yet it was in the New World that a dairy farmer's son called Frederick Banting had dreamed a dream and discovered insulin.

The experiments had been carried out in a small Canadian city called Toronto, situated by a lake described as "almost like an ocean,"

That however, is not the end of the journey of diabetes or the travels of insulin. In fact it may be called the beginning of another journey, the journey of "modern insulin".

Like the prophet in ancient times, standing on the summit of Mount Nebo near the Dead Sea, and like a modern scientist atop a summit overlooking the Pacific Ocean whom you will meet soon, you will need to imagine scaling a mountain to catch a glimpse of what lies ahead.

Since its discovery in Toronto in 1921 and the beginning of its use from 1922 in patients with diabetes, insulin had been made from the pancreases of pigs and cattle.

It is interesting to read the reaction of Dennis Kleid, one of the scientists involved in developing modern insulin, to the traditional production of insulin when in 1978, he toured a factory in Indiana, USA. where insulin was being made from pigs and cattle.

"There was a line of train cars filled with frozen pancreases." The process of producing insulin, according to the old methods being used by pharmaceutical companies like Lilly involved harvesting the pancreatic glands from animals. What struck the young scientist was the economy of scale.

23,500 animals had to be sacrificed in order to obtain around 8000 pounds of the gland. Then, using the traditional methods of making insulin, the 8000 pounds of pancreas yielded just one pound of the hormone.

Lilly which was the leading pharmaceutical company making insulin at that time sacrificed 56 million animals every year to satisfy the needs of patients with diabetes in the United States alone.

Clearly, there was a need to find a new source of insulin or develop another method of producing it.

The critical discovery which proved to be a magic wand for modern insulin has its beginnings in the work of a scientist called Paul Berg.

The journey of modern insulin begins with him.

The story of modern insulin is a story of confluence and cooperation, of competition and conflict, of pioneers and prophets, of young men and old.

It is also of the story of remarkable women whose brilliance was recognised albeit after a struggle but who will occupy seats in the highest levels of human accomplishment.

One truth is pre-eminent.

No one branch of science can claim primacy.

Modern insulin owes its birth to several branches of learning and the cooperation of many scientists in different disciplines.

An understanding of three commonly used scientific terms will make this part of the insulin's journey easier to follow.

Firstly, *heredity*.

This refers to passing on physical and mental characteristics from one generation to the next. For example, hair colour or the colour of eyes in a child may have been inherited from the father or mother.

The second term is *gene*.

A gene is the basic unit of heredity.

Modern insulin is the result of research into the way genes work. Research enabled scientists to change the makeup of genes and produce combinations of different genes. The combination of two hitherto distinctly different and independent genes (because they came from different organisms), is described by a word which was coined by one of the pioneers of this branch of science as is described below.

Thirdly, the word *recombinant* coined by Paul Berg who pioneered the technique refers to a combination of two unrelated organisms such as bacteria and a virus to produce a new organism which is a combination of the two. This had never been done before and was considered impossible until Berg's experiments proved otherwise. This revolutionary technique was used to produce the modern insulin which is now used by the millions of patients with diabetes around the world. This breakthrough pioneered *biotechnology* which has revolutionised the manufacture of insulin, and through it the treatment of diabetes.

At the time of Berg's experiments, the word *biotechnology* had not made it into the Oxford dictionary

The beginning of the story of modern insulin can be divided into three parts.

Firstly, the actual nature of the hormone insulin was clarified by the work of the English biochemist Frederick Sanger, whose painstaking – some would say back-breaking – research which took 12 years of solitary effort, demonstrated that insulin was a protein made up of individual units called amino acids which (in insulin) exist in a precise order called *sequence.*

Secondly, a new tool called *crystallography* enabled a woman called Dorothy Hodgkin to reveal the actual make-up (structure) of insulin.

Thirdly, a new method of measurement devised by two scientists in United States revolutionised the methods of conducting experiments which provided further useful and hitherto unknown facts such as the forms in which insulin existed in the human body. A physician, Solomon Berson, and a nuclear physicist Roslyn Yalow discovered this method called *radioimmunoassay.* They used this method to measure minute quantities of substances such as insulin in the blood.

The concept of modern insulin pioneered by Paul Berg's remarkable research would not have been possible without the aforementioned advances.

A further critical contribution which bridged the gap between the earlier understanding and knowledge and the findings of Berg's experiments was made through research carried out by two scientists called Frederick Griffiths in England and Oswald Avery in the United States.

In essence, the work of Griffith and Avery brought genes into the realm of molecular chemistry.

The details of these studies and discoveries provide an important background to Paul Berg's research and are presented before embarking on a description of Berg's experiments.

48

A QUIET ENGLISHMAN AND A QUIETER AMERICAN

Frederick Griffith's and Oswald Avery's Early Studies in the Development of Modern Insulin.

> *"The plans of the structures of nature are locked in the atoms themselves. From them alone, and from what they contain, grows infinite variety of the world".*
>
> Sir William Henry Bragg in *Concerning The Nature Of Things.* 1925.

Frederick Griffith (1877–1941).

It is a remarkable fact that the beginning of the journey of modern insulin began at around the same time as that of the Toronto team whose work delivered insulin for the treatment of diabetes in 1922. Many useful findings from experiments carried out during and in the period which followed the end of hostilities in World War One contributed to knowledge which helped the ongoing search for the nature of insulin.

Unlike Banting's quest, modern insulin's early history began with an entirely unrelated focus. And unlike Banting's bull-at-the gate approach and his single-minded pursuit of insulin, the celebrated experiments to be described here were carried out without any fanfare. The first series of experiments were done by a bacteriologist called Frederick Griffith.

Frederick Griffiths was an Englishman who, after graduating with a medical degree from Liverpool University and clinical training at the Liverpool Royal Infirmary, was employed as a bacteriologist by the Royal Commission on Tuberculosis. He was a loner who lived in a small house in Brighton but spent much of his time in a small apartment situated close to the laboratory where he worked.

When World War I broke out, Griffith's laboratory was taken over by the government and became the Ministry of Health's Bacteriological Laboratory with Griffiths as its medical officer. He already had an established reputation in the field of bacteriology, especially in infections caused by germs (bacteria). At the time Griffiths was working on the pneumococcus, the germ which had killed some 20 million men and women around the world. In the 1914 -18 war death from pneumonia which frequently followed as a complication of the flu had caused the death of more servicemen than had the war itself.

His critical contribution to the insulin story was that genetic material could be transferred between unrelated bacteria.

Starting with a large number of samples of this germ, Griffith searched for patterns of pneumonia as was common practice in such studies. He used mice as his experimental animals.

Working with two strains of pneumococcus – one with a smooth coat which caused the infection, and the other with a rough coat which was harmless – Griffith demonstrated that the characteristic in bacteria (in this case the pneumococcus) which caused the infection could be transferred from one strain to the other. In scientific jargon the transfer of the characteristics of one type of bacteria to an unrelated type is called *transformation.*

This phenomenon of transferring the characteristics or attributes from one type of bacteria to another was, to put it mildly, revolutionary. At that time – the early 1920s – the chemistry of such organisms was in its infancy.

The diminutive, unassuming Englishman published his findings in the *Journal of Hygiene, Volume 27, 113–159, 1928* with the title *The Significance of Pneumococcal Types.*

To say that the scientific word was stunned, would be an understatement.

At that time, molecular chemistry hardly existed as a subject. Nor was it pursued in any systematic way in research laboratories.

Many regarded Griffith's work as the first step in what developed as a widely practised discipline in research laboratories around the world.

Others went further, saying that the discovery led to the eventual "cracking of the code" and culminated several decades later, in the synthesis of insulin in the laboratory.

Disinclined to seek publicity, let alone prominence, Griffiths made no attempt to trumpet his success. The article detailed his work on the basis of which Griffiths concluded that he had "manipulated the immunologic specificity in pneumococci."

The claim left the scientific world speechless. Mukherjee stated that Griffiths' experiments had "launched the molecular biology revolution".

The work can be summarised in four steps as follows:

Firstly, Griffiths killed the infected, smooth strain bacteria with heat and injected the material into mice. The injections had no effect.

Secondly, he combined the material of the dead strain, which was no longer lethal, with the 2nd "rough "strain which had been harless on its own.

Thirdly, after mixing the dead smooth strain with the rough strain he injected the mixture into mice. The mice died.

Fourthly, Griffith examined the dead mice and made the astounding discovery that the "rough strain" pneumococcus had actually changed to the "smooth strain" variety.

His conclusion was that contact with material from the deadly smooth strain had changed the previously harmless, rough strain pneumococcus to the lethal smooth variety.

At the risk of dwelling on this, Griffiths' experiment had, for the first time, shown that the dead material from the smooth strain, although in itself "innocuous" having been killed by heat, could by simply being in contact with the hitherto harmless "rough strain" change the latter into the lethal "smooth strain" pneumococcus.

In scientific jargon this process of change in the smooth and rough strain pneumococci shown by Griffith's work is referred to as the principle of *transformation*.

A Very Private American Immigrant Scientist.

Oswald Avery (1877–1955).

The confirmation and further elucidation of Griffith's work came from a man born in the same year who, although of English heritage, was born in Halifax, Nova Scotia. His father Joseph Avery, a Baptist minister had emigrated from Britain in 1873. Initially they had lived in Halifax, Nova Scotia but in 1887 when he was ten, the family emigrated to the United States.

Oswald Avery, a quiet almost secretive individual was to write an equally critical second chapter in the insulin story started by Frederick Griffith.

The Protestant principles of the Baptist faith were inculcated in young Oswald from childhood and he remained a devout Christian to the end of his life.

Three years after graduating in medicine Oswald Avery switched to medical research. In 1913 he was appointed to the Rockefeller Hospital by Rufus Cole, Director of the Rockefeller Institute Hospital, where Avery remained for the rest of his professional life.

Whether or not Avery was sceptical of Griffiths' findings is unclear but it is part of the record of his work is that he repeated the Englishman's experiments before accepting the conclusions. More importantly, during these experiments Avery also identified the nature of the transforming substance.

The critical finding of this experiment was that the transforming material was Deoxyribonucleic Acid better known as DNA.

So it was DNA which had carried out the "transformation" described by Griffith.

This was the essential component of the gene which Avery recognised was responsible for making "predictable and hereditary" changes in cells.

It is an interesting historical fact that Avery's findings were published in 1944, in the middle of the Second World War (1939–1945), 14 years after Griffith's paper, which had been the result of work commissioned to address problems caused by pneumococcal infection which had decimated thousands of men and women serving in the armed forces during World War I as well as large numbers of the population in Europe including England.

In someways both Griffith's and Avery's work could be seen as going back to the basic nature of the cell and crossing traditional boundaries in different branches of science - physics, chemistry, biology- as had been created for the convenience of studying different aspects of the same problem. Already the chemistry of living things had given rise to the comparatively new science of biochemistry. Biology was being looked at through different disciplines with the use of technology – biotechnology.

The making of modern insulin is an example of this emerging branch of science.

It bears repeating that Griffith had discovered this in the early 1920s, when the chemistry of living organisms was very much in its infancy.

Thus while Frederick Banting, the discoverer of the "original" insulin was serving in the war, Griffith and Avery were labouring in the laboratory to add to the story of the hormone later isolated by the Canadian soldier.

Mukherjee in his book, *The Gene An Intimate History* hails Griffith's experiments as "the work that launched the molecular biology revolution."

Sir Peter Medawar (who in 1960 had shared the Nobel prize for Physiology or Medicine with the Australian Sir Frank McFarlane Burnett), was was equally effusive, declaring in his praise of Avery's discovery, that it was "the first step out of the dark ages of genetics."

The Nobel laureate Arne Tiselius referred to Avery as the most deserving scientist not to receive the Nobel Prize for his work even though he was nominated throughout the 1930s, 1940s and 1950s.

Griffith's experiments repeated by Avery led to the unlocking of one of the great mysteries of biology namely, the double helix of DNA. This much publicised work was carried out in 1953 in the Cavendish Laboratory in Cambridge by a team which included Francis Crick and James Watson who were later, awarded a share of the Nobel Prize.

Of particular interest in this account is that the head of the Cavendish Laboratory where this work was carried out by the Cambridge team, Sir William Lawrence Bragg, whom you met earlier as the 25-year-old winner of the Nobel Prize together with his father, Sir William Henry Bragg for their discovery of crystallography.

Many regards Griffith's work as the first step in the research which, several decades later, culminated in the synthesis of modern insulin.

The work of Griffith and Avery demonstrated an effect which is obvious in retrospect namely, that after being boiled the bacteria used by these workers had been turned into a solution. The solution was still able to transmit the genetic information from one strain to another. Therefore, many years later instead of treating the subject of his experiment as a virus, Berg the pioneer of recombinant technology, treated it as a chemical. He embarked on a series of experiments, with the aim of breaking open the gene, and "pasting" a piece of a gene from another virus to see if the new "combined" organism created would continue to work as it had previously. This had needed the development of a series of chemical reactions.

These stories serve to highlight the expertise of several researchers whose work contributed to the essential early stages of what eventually lead to the development of modern insulin.

49

THE STUFF OF SCIENCE-FICTION IN INSULIN'S JOURNEY

Creation without Reproduction.

In her novel, *The God of Small Things*, Arundhati Roy draws the reader into seeing the importance of little things. She challenges the Indian patriarchal society which practises and preaches the superiority of its own established values. The novel illustrates the effect of little things as the essence of life and Roy uses this to question the monopoly appropriated by the accepted norms and mores which had held sway in her native land for hundreds of years.

The novel also highlights the importance of seemingly insignificant practices and details in life as holding hitherto unrecognised power and importance.

A similar sequence of events may be applied to insulin.

Earlier researchers had considered the remnants left after auto-digestion of the gland following tying off the pancreatic duct to be too small to be significant. Similarly, the small pieces of the pancreas discarded as offal were left on the floor of the abattoirs of the Davies Company in Toronto until Banting had shown that the very same, seemingly unimportant, pieces contained the lifesaving insulin.

Modern insulin highlights the details of even smaller "things" as revealed by the development of crystallography, electron microscopy and especially the discovery of radioimmunoassay.

Imagine then, the reaction of the practitioners of the accepted concepts of biology to the discovery by the son of a cloth merchant in Brooklyn, United States, claiming to create life in a test tube and bypassing the union of two sexes which had been the method – the only method – of reproduction for human evolution for millions of years.

The initial and later advances which were unleashed by this discovery were through the efforts, insight, vision, instincts and courage, of a young scientist of humble beginnings, the son of a cloth merchant.

His name was Paul Berg.

Berg's Early Years.

"By learning to manipulate genes experimentally, you could learn to manipulate organisms experimentally. And by mixing and matching with the use of gene-manipulation and gene-sequencing tools, a scientist could interrogate not just genetics but the whole universe of biology with a kind of experimental audacity that was unimaginable in the past."

Paul Berg (1926–2023).

Paul Berg was born and raised in Brooklyn, a densely populated part of New York City which was settled by a mix of northern Europeans, including Scandinavians, Dutch, Russian, French and English immigrants. They were hard-working newcomers to the New World who, in addition to their own industrious ways, used slave labour until it ended in 1827. Many had started off with limited financial resources, and had to rely on their own initiative. What they emphasised upon their children was to not only develop a strong work ethic, but also to be uncompromising in their pursuit of excellence in their chosen careers through education.

Berg was the eldest of three children. His parents were Russian Jews. His father Harry Bergsaltz, born in Belarus was a clothing manufacturer of Russian-Jewish ancestry who had immigrated with his wife Sarah and settled in Brooklyn where Paul, the eldest of three sons, was born in 1926. He attended local schools.

A childhood interest in chemistry was to eventually culminate in his work on the structure of proteins in the 1950s. In his acceptance speech at the Nobel awards Berg said that a laboratory technician at Abraham Lincoln High School in the Brighton beach area of Brooklyn where he had been a student had fired his passion for discovery. Her name was Sophie Wolfe. The young woman had run a popular after-school biology club. Her method of teaching was to encourage the students to develop ways of finding answers to questions using their own initiative. The same young woman had also inspired Arthur Kornberg who had later befriended and mentored Berg at Stanford. Kornberg himself was a Nobel Laureate having won the award for Physiology or Medicine in 1959.

When he graduated from high school in January 1943 Berg wanted to join the war effort as a fighter pilot but was rejected and enlisted in the Navy at the age of 17. He worked as a submariner until discharged in 1946 when he returned to his biochemistry course at Penn State, graduating in 1948.

For his doctoral research at Western Reserve University (now Case Western Reserve University) in Cleveland, Ohio, Berg solved an important problem by demonstrating how Vitamin B 12 and folic acid enabled animals to make the amino acid methionine. This was the beginning of his interest in the study of enzymes.

It was at this point in his career that Berg had met Arthur Kornberg who was to have a profound influence on him. Berg worked in Kornberg's laboratory at Washington University School of Medicine in St Louis in 1953–1954.

Kornberg, the 1959 Nobel Laureate who had discovered the enzyme (DNA polymerase) which is essential for making, rearranging, and repairing DNA remained a strong influence Berg's academic life. Later, this class of enzymes formed the basis of the discovery of recombinant DNA by Paul Berg, which started the biotechnology revolution.

Kornberg and Berg had similar backgrounds. They were children of immigrant parents who had to work hard to make ends meet. Both had the value of education impressed upon them since childhood. Kornberg's father, Joseph had worked in a sweatshop as a sewing machine operator for nearly 30 years. Although he had no formal education, Joseph Kornberg spoke six languages.

A period of intensive research in various centres, including Washington University School of Medicine and Cambridge in England preceded Berg's tenure at Stanford University in 1959.

In 1959 Kornberg moved most of the Washington University department, including Berg, to a new biochemistry department situated in Stanford University School of Medicine where Berg stayed for the rest of his life.

50

A GLIMPSE FROM THE MOUNTAIN TOP

Berg's "What if" Moment.
A World War II Veteran's Contribution to Modern Insulin.

Renato Dulbecco (1914–2012) was an Italian scientist, who had spent his academic life studying viruses which by infecting animal cells, cause cancers. He, like Frederick Banting, was a veteran though in Dulbecco's case it was the Second World War (1939–1945), when he had fought in France and Russia. And, like Banting, the discoverer of insulin, Dulbecco had also been wounded in action and hospitalised.

After the war, Dulbecco joined the Resistance against German occupation but later had left Italy for the United States where he had worked in different universities to continue his experiments on animal viruses and bacteria.

Dulbecco worked at the Salk Institute which sits atop a hill overlooking the waters of the Pacific Ocean.

In 1967–68 Paul Berg spent 11 months at the Salk Institute on sabbatical leave. It was here in 1967 that the 41 year old biochemist working in a laboratory on the summit of a mountain in California glimpsed in his imagination a biological landscape unlike any other in recorded history and the thought of crossing biological boundaries which had been in place since the beginning of human history occurred to him.

While working with the Italian scientist Berg had become interested in the transmission of information from the cells of bacteria to viruses and his interest had shifted from studying protein synthesis to the study of animal viruses especially a virus called SV 40. He was intrigued and astonished by the capability of this virus to enter infected cells, then remain inactive for long periods until activated.

In his time with Dulbecco Berg had been accompanied by his longtime research assistant Marianne Dieckmann. In the Salk Institute's virology laboratory Berg and Dieckmann learned how to work with simian virus 40 (SV40).

Always with his finger on the pulse of progress in research in his field, Berg quickly recognised an opportunity when, in the early 1970s work with DNA had advanced to the stage of the protein being manipulated. He seized on the opportunity to attempt to join the DNA of SV 40 to the DNA of bacteria or bacterial viruses. His success in this exercise resulted in hybrid or chimeric molecules later to be known as *recombinant* molecules, the term he himself had coined.

What if the SV 40 virus could be equipped with genes which could be placed inside the cells of human beings who would then be carrying new hereditary information?

Such questions were uppermost in Berg's mind when he returned to Stanford, and told his friend and mentor Kornberg of his experience during his sabbatical.

Kornberg was ambivalent about Berg pursuing his work on genes. But Berg could not get the idea out of his head and Kornberg was unable to persuade his young associate to give up on that area of research.

Berg had seen before anyone else, the possibility of artificially engineering a foreign gene.

51

BERG'S DREAM. THE CONCEPT OF MODERN INSULIN

"The future belongs to those who believe in the beauty of their dreams."

Eleanor Roosevelt.

Unlike Banting, who had limited experience and expertise in research but whose dream had led to the discovery of insulin in 1921, Berg was a mature, highly qualified and respected scientist at this stage of his career. What he had in common with Banting was a "dream" – a vision as we have called it here, but one which, like Banting's dream, would not go away inspite of his senior colleague and mentor Kornberg's reservations.

Returning to Stanford after his sabbatical with Dulbecco, Berg devised and refined a method for "cutting" genes, then joining ("stitching") them. In technical jargon this is called *"splicing"*- the two pieces forming a new piece which had been cut from a gene from a different organism.

He had then led a team of scientists to eventually combine genetic material from viruses with the DNA of bacteria. The essence of bergs groundbreaking experiments are described below.

Scientists who work with bacteria and viruses had been engaged in the workings of these organisms since the 1960s, and had shown that each of these organisms had it own tools for different purposes. Cells need special enzymes to repair damaged parts. Such enzymes allow the cell to replace the damaged part with a new piece of DNA. For this purpose, there are different enzymes for cutting and different enzymes for pasting. Since this is a normal happening in the life of bacteria and viruses, the question was whether a piece of one could be pasted into the other and still retain its ability to work as it had originally.

Berg's fame is due to his experiment which demonstrated that this was achievable. In the course of doing the experiments on this subject he had also discovered and developed methods of cutting and joining pieces of DNA.

In 1971 Berg and David Jackson, a post-doctoral researcher in his laboratory, developed an effective method for doing the landmark gene-splicing experiment which was an essential preliminary step in recombinant DNA technology. Using certain enzymes they succeeded in removing pieces of DNA which interrupted the sequence of genes, then joining the two remaining sections of DNA thus creating the first molecule from the DNA of two different species, one was a virus and the other a bacterium.

When he saw what he had managed to achieve in a test tube, the realisation dawned on him that what had actually been accomplished was the creation of a unique *biological* phenomenon *artificially*.

This previously unknown technique had succeeded in combining / joining two unrelated organisms. Berg coined the term *recombinant* for this new technique. The word had not existed until that time.

To describe Berg's work as groundbreaking would be an understatement. At that time the word *biotechnology* had not even made it into the Oxford English dictionary.

For his revolutionary discovery, Berg won the 1980 Nobel Prize for Chemistry. The award was shared with Walter Gilbert and Frederick Sanger who had worked in a related field. Their contributions will be described later in this account.

Berg's method which was later used by Cohen and Boyer in experiments which culminated in the creation of modern insulin has become part of the folklore of biotechnology.

The seminal experiments which led to the birth of a new technology are now referred to as genetic engineering or gene manipulation.

Modern insulin is a product of genetic engineering.

Berg was perhaps not unaware of the wider implications of the work he was doing. He realised that genes could be combined and altered by cutting and pasting, then moved from one organism to another.

This included the possibility of moving a piece of an animal DNA to a virus and, wait for it, to *human* DNA.

At the risk of overemphasising the point, the human gene could be put inside the cells of bacteria.

Methods to achieve this combination between different organisms had been known for some years, but what was novel was it's application in the way Berg envisioned it.

Summarising Berg's work as described here runs the risk of giving the impression that firstly, it was simple and, secondly, it was easily accomplished.

Such assumptions, if made, are incorrect.

Every step required important contributions by different associates in Berg's laboratory as well as cooperation with, and assistance from, other scientists.

The initial experiments began in Berg's laboratory with help from a postdoctoral researcher called David Jackson. It is interesting to come across critical pieces of information, provided generously by other scientists who made time to help colleagues even though they themselves had their own projects to attend to. This in fact, is what happened in the very first part of Berg's work with Jackson. In the same institution there was a graduate student called Peter Lobban who had come to Stanford from MIT and was pursuing his own project. Yet Lobban always made time to provide technical advice to Peter Jackson.

Berg's new "creation" had been made in a test tube. It was a new life which had been made without the biologic process of reproduction which been the only way new life had been created during millions of years of human evolution.

At the time, the new method of producing the combination of a virus with bacteria did not have a name and, as noted above, the word *recombinant* was coined by Berg. These experiments marked the beginnings of biotechnology.

For the purposes of this narrative, there's another important reason to record that an enzyme which had contributed to the success of Janet Mertz's experiment in Berg's laboratory in late 1972 had been supplied by Professor Herbert Boyer, a pioneer in the development and production of modern insulin. Boyer's role in the insulin story will be detailed later.

Berg's work, which can be summarised as the successful insertion of a piece of DNA from the bacterium E. coli into the DNA of an animal virus (SV 40) was a milestone in science and, as mentioned above, won him the Nobel Prize for Chemistry in 1980.

Unlike the furore which followed the awarding of the Nobel Prize for the discovery of insulin by Banting, there were no dissenting voices when Berg's work was recognised by the same award.

Yet some critical parts of the experiment which eventually resulted in the creation of the recombinant molecule had been achieved through help from other scientists in Berg's laboratory as well as others who were pursuing their own research. Berg was always aware of the contribution, not only from members of his own team but also from other colleagues and acknowledge this in his acceptance speech in the ceremonies of the Nobel award.

The cooperation and contributions of his younger associates was reflected in the names listed as authors of Berg's classical paper which announced the recombinant technique to the scientific world.

D. A. Jackson, RH Symons, P.Berg: *Biochemical method for inserting new genetic information into DNA of Simian Virus 40. Circular SV40 DNA molecules containing lambda phage genes and the galactose operon of Escherichia coli. Proceedings National Academy Sci. USA, 69, 2904–2909 (1972).*

Author's apology.

"Circular molecules? lambda phage genes? operon?"

"Hold it right there", I hear you saying, and I agree. If you, gentle reader, found in the title of the paper, terms which are strange to you, let me reassure you that they were new to me also. Chemistry as taught in medical school at the University of Sydney (Australia) when I was there in the late 1950s and early 1960s as well as in the later years when I engaged in further studies, had not advanced to anywhere near the levels reached just 20 years later.

Try to be patient with yourself – and with me – because the story as its unfolds in my telling keeps technical terms to the bare minimum.

It is important to remind ourselves of the work that had been done by earlier workers and which eventually lead to the development of modern insulin.

The experiments carried out by Griffith and Avery had demonstrated that the bacteria they used had in fact been boiled and turned into a solution, which to their surprise, was still able to transmit the genetic information from one strain to another.

Based on their findings Berg, instead of treating the subject of his experiment as a virus, treated it as a chemical. He embarked on a series of experiments with the aim of breaking open the gene and "pasting" a piece of a gene from another virus to see if the new "combined" organism created would continue to work as it had previously. This needed the development of a series of chemical reactions.

An observer soon comes comes to realise that the contribution of several researchers was needed in virtually every step in the development of modern insulin before the finished product was obtained.

Today, we hear of insulin having been "cloned" in bacteria. Cloning is the term used to describe a process of making identical copies of a particular piece of DNA.

In the case of insulin, cloning permitted the making of insulin by bacteria.

These experiments marked the beginning of biotechnology which was to eventually result in making insulin in a test tube.

An interesting and important incident in this early stage of the narrative is about an enzyme which was essential to the success of Berg's and Jackson's work.

As had been mentioned by Berg himself, many of the steps of the process of cutting and pasting DNA were extremely tedious. Berg had called that part of the exercise "a biochemist's nightmare."

In late 1972, Janet Mertz, a graduate student who was helping Berg, had also come to a dead end in her search for a way to shorten the process.

Then, by chance she found out that a professor of microbiology in San Francisco had developed a particular enzyme which could be used to cut DNA. The enzyme, called EcoRI would reduce the process of cutting and pasting DNA from six steps to two which would decidedly provide a solution to the tedious process.

Berg was delighted.

> "Janet really made the process vastly more efficient. Now, in just a few chemical reactions, we could generate new pieces of DNA… She cut them, mixed them, added an enzyme that could join ends to ends, and then showed that she had gotten a product that shared the properties of both the starting materials."

Who was the generous professor who supplied the essential agent,?
Herb Boyer.

Remember him because he becomes an increasingly prominent presence in the story of the development of recombinant "modern insulin".

As will be seen on more than one occasion in this account, Boyer was known for his friendliness when it came to sharing his findings and experimental materials with colleagues, a trait which is not always seen in the competitive, sometimes cut-throat, research environment.

Boyer's engaging personality and his sense of humour coupled with the gift of being able to make complicated scientific information understandable for lay people, may well make him a favourite of many readers of this book.

You will get to know him better.

52

WHEN ALL HELL BROKE LOOSE

Early Hurdles for the "New Age Scientists".

The hopes and fears of all the years…
Phillips Brooks 1868.

In June 1972, Janet Mertz went from Berg's laboratory in Stanford to Cold Spring Harbour in New York to attend a short course on animal cells and viruses. When she described her plans to make chimeras from virus and bacterial cells, then propagate the combination in bacterial cells, all hell broke loose.

Not only students, but several senior scientists who were there as advisors and supervisors assailed Mertz with question after question mostly about the central issue of the uncertainty of the nature of the combination described. What were the possible consequences of letting loose such unique and previously non-existent "creatures" on the human population etc. etc.?

One of the instructors in the course called Berg directly regarding the dangers of crossing "evolutionary boundaries. The virus "SV 40" being used by Berg was known to cause tumours in hamsters but the risks to humans were not known at that time ie the 1970s. E.coli is quite a common inhabitant of the gut of human beings. Could the combination of the virus and the bacteria cause cancers in human beings? The repercussions of such questions were to have a profound effect on the pursuit of modern insulin. We will return to this important story shortly.

Whether or not Berg had harboured private reservations about the wider implications and repercussions of recombinant technology while engaged in his experiments is unclear. Although concerned after hearing of Mertz's experience he still considered that the risks were minimal.

He was to question that view a few months later when in the summer of 1972 he was invited to conduct a seminar in Erice, an ancient town situated near the western coast of Sicily.

Speaking to a group of some 80 graduate students Berg presented his data on the chimera experiments produced through the recombinant technique.

To quote Mukherjee who, being a student in Berg's laboratory at that time, was in an ideal position to follow the unfolding saga,

"the students were electrified." Berg was assailed with questions as he had expected, but the direction of the conversation surprised him. In Janet Mertz's presentation at Cold Spring Harbour in 1971, the biggest concern had been safety. There she was asked how she guarantee that their genetic chimeras would not unleash biological chaos on humans? In Sicily, by contrast the conversation had turned quickly to politics, culture, and ethics. Berg was bombarded with questions on the possible implications for humans and human societies?"

Whether or not Berg had contemplated such reactions to his work is unclear. However, he quickly realised that he could not ignore the possibility of the concerns which had been raised in the two meetings leading to further, more widespread repercussions. He could not ignore the possibility of the wider community beyond that of scientists being concerned, even fearing what his research could lead to. Berg would have been aware of the public perception of strange creatures from another world as had been described by Michael Crichton in science fiction novels.

Michael Crichton (1942–2008), a Doctor with a Fertile Imagination.

In 1969 Michael Crichton aged twenty-seven, a Harvard medical graduate who was already better known for his imaginative novels and films, wrote *The Andromeda Strain.* The science-fiction novel described a deadly germ which had come from outer space to infect people in Arizona. Given the popularity of Crichton's writing and later, the films based on his books including *Jurassic Park,* it is tempting to speculate that the students listening to Berg imagined a similar scenario being created through the recently developed genetic engineering and recombinant technology being described by the Stanford University professor.

This was before the film had shown the phantasmagoric images created from *Jurassic Park* (published in 1990) which was described as a "cautionary tale about genetic engineering."

But there was enough in Chrichton's earlier work, including *The Andromeda Strain* to fire the imagination especially of the young.

After all, Berg had used bacterial strains in his experiments. That such fears were not restricted to the young came out in the Asilomar meetings which are described below.

53

THE ATOMIC BOMB AND EINSTEIN IN THE INSULIN STORY

This interesting chapter in the modern insulin story follows Berg's attempt to reach out to his fellow-scientists and researchers through two conferences, known as the Asilomar meetings which he arranged.

The Asilomar Meetings.

Clearly the reactions of the young people in the seminar at Erice had concerned Berg. That, together with questions raised by many in the scientific community and concerns expressed by some sections of the community led to Berg organising a conference in California to address the issues associated with the emerging technologies, he was pioneering.

The meetings were held in Monterey, a city on California's Central Coast which used to be popular with fishermen. It is described in John Steinbeck's novel *Cannery Row* which contains memorable passages on the Great Depression and how it affected the sardine fishing industry in Monterey. In recent years Asilomar has become a popular tourist resort because of the ocean front and it's beach of white sand.

There were two Asilomar meetings. The first referred to as Asilomar 1 was held in 1974.

Scientists from various related disciplines including biochemists, molecular biologists (like Boyer), and experts on genetics and viruses participated to discuss concerns about the new technologies and laboratory methods being employed to study genes.

Apart from providing information to the different groups of researchers on progress being made by other laboratories, little came out of this first meeting except for what has become known as the "Berg letter."

It spoke of scientists voluntarily deferring further experimentation with recombinant material until the potential hazards had been examined and effective methods to prevent the spread of such material were developed.

In 1974, Paul Berg wrote an article which was published in highly respected scientific publications including *Nature, Science* and *Proceedings of the National Academy of Sciences.* The article sent ripples around the globe especially in scientific circles. The only consensus, if any, was for caution. Some scientists even suggested deferring genetic experiments until the risks had been identified and addressed.

However, these issues did not discourage all the scientists involved in genetic experiments.

From the point of view of the development of modern insulin, Boyer and Cohen had continued their work despite the controversy swirling around them.

A second meeting - Berg called it Asilomar 2 - was organised and chaired by Berg and Maxine Singer, a molecular biologist and administrator. It was held in February 1975.

This time a group of prominent scientists, including Paul Berg, Singer and Sydney Brenner, (also a molecular biologist), drafted a document containing specific recommendations.

The document stated that *"the new techniques, which permit combination of genetic information from very different organisms, place us in an area of biology with many unknowns… it is this ignorance that has compelled us to conclude that it would be wise to exercise considerable caution in performing this research."*

The recommendations were presented to the meeting on the final morning, and contrary to the expectations of those who had drafted the document, all the proposals were accepted.

Philippe Kourilsky, one of six invited French participants at the second conference commented that the participants did not include "ecologists with a normal point of view." He went on to say that he had found the conference exciting because of "the scale of this scientific adventure, the great expanses which had opened to research, and because no one could be indifferent to the debate over the power and responsibilities of scientists."

Kourilski also said that "on the frontiers of the unknown, the analysis of benefits and hazards were locked up in concentric circles of ignorance. How could one determine the reality without experimenting… without taking a minimum of risk?"

From the point of view of research on the subject, the result of the Asilomar meetings was to agree to a voluntary moratorium on this aspect of research pending further discussions specifically on the risks and how they may be controlled.

As noted by Mukherjee, although the conference addressed the biological risks of gene cloning, the question of its ethics and moral implications remained unaddressed.

However, it had placed the studies on genes front and centre, not only in scientific deliberations, but also in public consciousness.

Mukherjee draws a parallel between the profound concern verging on fear of recombinant technology as existed at the time of the Asilomar conference in 1975 and the risks to humanity posed by the atomic bomb in the Second World War 1939–1945.

Einstein and Oppenheimer in the Insulin Story.

The writing of this book which I started in early 2023 coincided with the release later that year of Christopher Nolan's film *Oppenheimer* on the life of Robert Oppenheimer (1904–1967), a theoretical physicist largely remembered for his role in developing the atomic bomb. The film is an absorbing depiction of the development of the atomic bomb under the conflicted scientist's initiative, influence and guidance. The top-secret assignment was called the Manhattan Project.

The Manhattan Project.

Few historic incidents portray the drama including the fraught relationship between politics and science and the use of science and scientists by government and bureaucrats more dramatically – and tragically– than the development of the atomic bomb.

The top secret Manhattan Project was a joint operation of the American and British allies in World War II.

It is a part of history remembered by many of today's population, including those who were children, during the 1939 to 1945 period of World War II. The chief protagonists in the story of modern insulin namely, Paul Berg, Herb Boyer and Stan Cohen had also lived through World War II.

On August 6, 1945 an American B-29 bomber called *Enola Gay* piloted by Colonel Paul Warfield Tibbetts Jr. dropped the first atomic bomb dubbed *Little Boy* on the Japanese city of Hiroshima.

On August 9, 1945 Major Charles William Sweeney, pilot of *Bockscar* dropped an atomic bomb dubbed *Fat Man,* on Nagasaki.

The bombings resulted in the death of 250,000 people including children, but the final figure for deaths and disfigurement ran into the millions.

As recorded and detailed in the Potsdam Declaration, Japan surrendered the following day, August 10,1945.

In Nolan's film, the assignment of priority in the research on the atomic bomb is highlighted by the appointment of the overseer/administrator of the project. It wasn't a scientist but a high-ranking soldier, Brigadier General Leslie Groves. In the film the role is played by Matt Damon, (the hero Jason Bourne in many Robert Ludlum movies).

Two elements in the film reminded me of a parallel between Oppenheimer's work and the discovery and development of the recombinant technology used in producing modern insulin.

In an early scene in the film when atomic energy was in its infancy, Oppenheimer was asked if he could "hear the music" of the possibilities of atomic energy. He could.

Berg also, like a biblical prophet and a modern-day martyr, had envisioned a previously unknown possibility of combining two entirely unrelated living organisms and creating a unique, artificial "life".

Later, Oppenheimer was conflicted when the possibilities of adverse consequences of his invention became the subject of worldwide publicity on the news and film-clips. Unlike Berg who had also agonised over possible conflicts inherent in recombinant technology, at least some of Berg's scientific colleagues had provided support. Oppenheimer, on the other hand, experienced the loneliness of rejection by those who were, as shown in the film, the decision-makers in the project.

The physicist's contribution to science after the Manhattan project was not shown in the film.

Albert Einstein Writes to President Roosevelt.

The letter written in August 1939, though signed by Einstein, had not been written by him but by Leo Szilard (1898–1964). Szilard had discovered and patented the nuclear chain reaction in the early 1930s. In the letter, the two scientists cautioned Roosevelt against the potential of nuclear energy "for construction of bombs" which they warned had the capacity to destroy whole cities. This was the letter that led to the formation of the powerful Advisory Committee on Uranium in 1942, and ultimately to the creation of the atomic bomb through the advice of another physicist, J.Robert Oppenheimer.

As described above the atomic bomb dropped on the Japanese cities. Nagasaki and Hiroshima effectively ended the Second World War.

Oppenheimer, derided because of the devastation caused by the atomic bomb, was nevertheless a brilliant physicist and teacher. An oft-quoted advice to his students was that articles written in the scientific literature should be read in their original language. Had Banting and Best, whose work preceded Oppenheimer's controversial contributions, been familiar with French and German or had access to translations, they would have gained valuable information on, and findings related to, earlier research on insulin by European scientists particularly Nikolai Paulesco and, closer to home, the experiments of Israel Kleiner at the Rockefeller Institute in New York.

Kleiner's research is included in this work to describe in greater detail the research on insulin which he had done before the experiments carried out by Banting and Best.

It is interesting that Macleod had commented on Kleiner's research in his letter to the Banting and Best while he (Macleod) had been on holidays. One can only assume that in the euphoria of having discovered that their extract and succeeded in lowering the blood glucose levels in the dogs, the two Toronto workers had not followed up on Macleod's comment. Neither for that matter, had Macleod.

Both the First World War (1914–1918), and the Second World War (1939–1945) feature in the insulin stories. Firstly, the animal-sourced hormone was discovered and isolated by Frederick Banting on his return from war service in France in 1918. Secondly, modern insulin owed its development to the work of several scientists and physicians starting with the work of Frederick Griffiths in London which was part of the war effort in Britain, also in the First World War. Paul Berg had served in the submarines during World War II and had resumed his studies after the war in 1946.

The "fear factor" generated by Berg's recombinant experiments, spread far and wide, including in the public sphere. His personal role in this difficult period included writing to a wide constituency in order to explain the technology in the hope of explaining the technology and the cautious approach of the scientists.

A letter to a local politician who was vehemently opposed to the recombinant experiments is reproduced in order to illustrate Berg's approach to the challenge of working with authorities at various levels of government as well as private organisations.

The mayor of Cambridge (Massachusetts) features later in this work in the drama of the race to develop modern insulin.

I found online the letter Paul Berg wrote to Alfred Velluchi, mayor of Cambridge, Massachusetts where both Harvard University and the Massachusetts Institute of Technology (MIT) are located.

It is reproduced to provide an insight into the approach taken by Berg to allay the fears of leaders in the community.

Paul Berg's letter to Alfred Vellucci Mayor of Cambridge, Massachusetts.

July 2, 1976.

Paul Berg,
Professor of Biochemistry.
Department of Biochemistry,
Stanford University Medical Centre,
Stanford, California, 94305.

Honourable Mayor, Alfred E. Vellucci and the Honourable
City Council of Cambridge,
City Hall.
Cambridge, Massachusetts.

Gentlemen:
Having been a pioneer in developing the recombinant DNA methodology as well as a leader amongst the scientists who first expressed concern over the potential risks of this research, I feel obliged to comment on the discussions on this matter now before you.

Few scientists, anywhere, deny that recombinant DNA research will revolutionise our understanding of basic biological processes; and, there is little doubt that in time, this increased knowledge, will yield far- reaching benefits for medicine, industry, and agriculture. Admittedly, the pursuit of these goals carries with it potential risks, but irrespective of the claims made by the researchers and critics, the extent and the certainty of these risks are largely conjectural. And to state that the benefits are tenuous and hypothetical while the risks are real and immediate is to engage in sophistry bordering on dishonesty.

I believe that the recently, promulgated guidelines for recombinant DNA experimentation are more stringent than any scientific evidence indicates is needed to ensure safety. The required procedures are not "smoke screams"; physical containment was designed specifically to control accidental dispersal and human error, and there is documented experience by which to judge the efficacy of these facilities. Moreover, most experiments have an additional requirement which mandates the use of specially constructed organisms that cannot survive in natural environments. The two forms of containment complement each other and provide an effective barrier to dissemination of the experimental organisms.

There are those who propose a ban on this research because of the use of E. coli. These individuals advocate waiting until safer organisms are developed. But, predictions about the existence of rare and fastidious safer organisms that could replace E. coli are highly speculative. Most scientists who are familiar with the genetic chemistry of E. coli believe that the effective biological containment can be achieved by such specially modified organisms.

Many scientists and laymen alike are deeply concerned that the Cambridge City Council is considering suppression of a serious and responsible search for new knowledge. The implications of such actions are ominous indeed. What additional forms of legitimate and worthy inquiry – scientific, artistic, or political – will-self appointed vigilante groups next condemn on the pretext of imagined risks? Consider carefully which people certain scientists speak for, and whose message they carry.

An alternate to suppression is cooperation. Would it not make more sense for the Cambridge City Council to join with its responsible scientific community in efforts to monitor compliance with the guidelines, and ensure the safety of the scientists and the public at large? Such an action could lead to a partnership for progress, rather than a conspiracy of repression. Cooperative ventures might even alleviate the traditional tensions of the town-gown relationship.

I am hopeful, yes, even optimistic, that you will hear reason, not rhetoric, and act wisely rather than precipitously.

Respectfully,
Paul Berg (signature)

54

BERG A WOUNDED SCIENTIST?

Berg returned to his research activities after the development of recombinant technology, but his output was diminished. I searched for written material on this part of Berg's career, but failed to find any information in the literature.

A question which in my reading has received scant attention in medical and scientific literature is the effect of the various aspects of the controversy over recombinant technology on Berg himself.

Preserved as the Berg Papers in the NIH collection is a brief chronology of his work which is reproduced here.

1952–1959 Classical Biochemistry to Molecular Biology.
1959–1975 Tumour Viruses and Recombinant Technology.
1973–1980 Recombinant Technology. Researchers' Responsibilities.
1980 – Onwards. Changing Academic Landscape.

One cannot help noticing that after the Asilomar meetings (1974–75) there appears to have been a decided fall in Berg's scientific/research output even though he is said to have remained active in research until 2000. I could find no reference in the literature on the emotional trauma inflicted on Berg through the arguments for and against his discovery of recombinant technology.

There is little doubt that the sophisticated methodology in modern scientific research requires substantial expenditure on equipment, instruments, and materials, as well as salaries for highly skilled and qualified scientists. Apart from government, large pharmaceutical companies all over the world, are also investing substantial funds in the hope of developing and discovering effective treatments for diabetes.

One area in which cost considerations are seen clearly is the development of new medications for the treatment of diabetes. An inevitable consequence of such a development is the cost of drugs on the market, which is often beyond the means of the disadvantaged in the population, as well as entire communities in under-developed nations.

A good example of this is the publicity generated by a drug with the chemical name of *semaglutide* and brand names of *Ozempic* and *Wegovy* which, in addition to its effectiveness in treating Type 2 diabetes, also helps people who do not have diabetes to lose weight.

The popularity of the medication with non-diabetic individuals who could afford to buy the expensive drug "over the counter" without a doctor's prescription led to a shortage of supply in some countries for patients with diabetes.

Berg's Life after Asilomar.

Two aspects of the discovery of modern recombinant insulin have received scant attention.

Firstly, it brought back both biology and genetics to centre stage and secondly, it led to chemistry being expanded to *biochemistry* which in turn, through the remarkable progress in technology due to revolutionary innovations many of which followed Berg's pioneering studies, heralded the era of *biotechnology.*

Biotechnology was not only a new concept but a revolutionary one. The seminal experiments which led to the birth of a new technology are now referred to as genetic engineering or gene manipulation. Berg has been called the father of genetic engineering.

Modern insulin is a product of genetic engineering.

Paul Berg "live."

It is interesting to hear Berg's views on the controversy many years later. In a live interview I found online, he recalled that at least initially in the meetings in Asilomar, there was concern and fear amongst the scientists engaged in those experiments, of the risks of producing a new form of life through the recombinant technology. He said that the first meeting (in Asilomar) was to examine the dangers to the scientists themselves but in retrospect, the fear of such dangers were found to be spurious. Given Berg's clearly stated reservations on experiments using recombinant technology in the earlier period, it is interesting to hear the reaction of Boyer and Cohen recorded in the sections describing their findings. Both had continued their experiments to develop recombinant insulin in spite of the reservations expressed during Asilomar conferences.

According to David Baltimore's obituary on Berg, it was Boyer and Cohen's work on combining two molecules from different organisms as presented at a 1974 summer Gordon Research Conference that the attendees were concerned by the possible implications and had written a letter to the US National Academy of Sciences, calling for the potential hazards of the new technology to be examined.

This had been a reason for Berg to become involved in the controversy and organising the Asilomar conferences.

It is important to recognise that Boyer and Cohen were not the only scientists who had continued to use the recombinant technique during the voluntary, moratorium agreed to at Asilomar.

This brings us to the interesting story of another molecular chemist. Har Gobind Khorana at the Massachusetts Institute of Technology had also continued recombinant DNA research during the moratorium.

Har Gobind Khorana (1922–2011) "the Prodigy from Punjab."

The Nobel laureate in Physiology or Medicine in 1968, was born in India but had done his scientific research in USA, initially at the University of Wisconsin and later at the Massachusetts Institute of Technology. Khorana had devoted his life to the interpretation of the genetic code and it's role in protein synthesis.

Like Berg, Khorana had also needed a large team of scientists for his project which was to make an artificial gene. His experiments had needed "nine years of work by 24 postdoctoral fellows."

Khorana's contribution to the story of modern insulin is that one of his students Saran Narang had trained Keiichi Itakura who in turn had been head hunted by Art Riggs to join the City of Hope research team. Khorana had also influenced one of the teachers of David Goeddel, another "star" in the modern insulin story. Marvin Caruthers had worked with Khorana for five years before moving to take up the Professorship of Biochemistry at the University of Colorado at Boulder, where Goeddel had studied before moving to California to work for Genentech .

After the initial furore over recombinant DNA research, Berg remained involved in the controversy. He travelled throughout the United States, meeting with not only academic bodies such as university boards, but also City Councils to talk them out of putting obstacles in the way of recombinant DNA research.

For a particularly colourful incident involving Local Government officials you will later read about the battles between a Harvard professor and a politician in the form of the combative Cambridge (Massachusetts) City mayor Alfred Velluchi whom you have met already.

In the late 1980s, when there were heated discussions over starting the Human Genome Project largely because of calculations that had suggested the cost of it could be in the order of $3 billion, Berg had used his persuasive style to help get it launched. Eventually, the project was launched in 1990 and completed in 2003.

The human genome project, it could be argued, cost more in time, than in money. It took 13 years, and the cost at $2.7 billion was marginally less than the projected 3 billion. What it achieved however, was to start the age of genomics which enabled the scientific unravelling of many processes playing a role in genetic abnormalities which cause cancer and various inherited diseases.

A practical and widely used advance made possible by genomics was the at-home "RAT" (rapid antigen testing) kit which could be employed by individuals to detect the presence of Covid during the recent 2019 pandemic.

55

PAUL BERG NOBEL LAUREATE

There was no surprise – or dissent – when in 1980, Berg was awarded the Nobel Prize in Chemistry for "his fundamental studies on the biochemistry of nucleic acids, with particular regard to recombinant DNA."

If any, a surprise may have been that he shared the prize with Walter Gilbert and Frederick Sanger who were honoured for their work on sequences in nucleic acids (DNA and RNA).

Berg delivered the Nobel Lecture on December 8, 1980. He began with the following quotation, "Although we are sure not to know everything and rather likely not to know very much, we can know anything that is known to man, and may, with luck and sweat, even find out somethings that have not before been known to man."

The author of that quote was J. Robert Oppenheimer.

Given the trials and tribulations faced by Oppenheimer as described earlier, it's not hard to guess why Berg had chosen this quote. Berg's discovery which made possible the creation of life in a test tube and which bypassed the natural evolutionary method of reproduction had raised fundamental questions on the ethics of his experiments. He himself was very conscious of this and was instrumental in persuading the scientific community to exercise caution, even possibly imposing conditions and restrictions on the use of the recombinant technology he had pioneered.

Berg was highly respected and most (but not all) other scientists engaged in research on recombinant technology agreed to a voluntary moratorium on certain aspects of recombinant DNA research until the risks had been properly evaluated.

Furthermore, the conference which addressed these issues on recombinant DNA held in Asilomar in 1975 at which the potential hazards were discussed had set guidelines for biotechnology research. There was a careful evaluation of potential hazards referred to as the *precautionary principle.* Oppenheimer had wrestled with similar ethical questions himself when developing the atomic bomb.

Berg's lecture can be read in full online but it is important to recognise his gracious acknowledgement of the many associates, assistants and colleagues who had contributed to his success. Nor did he forget his indebtedness to those who had guided him in the early years of his career. The first to be mentioned was Arthur Kornberg, his friend and mentor who had brought Berg to Stanford University where the bulk of the work on recombinant technology had been carried out.

By nature, Berg was known as being cultured, friendly, interested in sport, art, music - and good food. In 1947 he had married Mildred Levy, a nurse and an amateur musician.

Berg never forgot his roots. His ancestors, as mentioned earlier, had been hard-working immigrants who had remained devoted to their Jewish faith. Berg remained a lifelong member of a Jewish fraternity which he had joined during his undergraduate years at Penn State University.

Berg retired in 2000 but kept in touch with scientific progress in his field through frequent meetings with his colleagues.

In addition to his numerous scientific articles Berg, with Maxine Singer, wrote several books on genetics for non-scientists. In 2003 they had worked together on a biography of the pioneering genetics expert George Beadle in *George Beadle: An Uncommon Farmer.*

In the epigram at the beginning of this piece on Paul Berg, he had spoken of *unimaginable experimental audacity*. There would be little argument that he himself also possessed – and retained – this rare quality.

Revealed! A Nobel Laureate's Secret Passion.

During the Vietnam War (1955 to 1975), Berg's biochemistry class at Stanford School of Medicine was extremely popular. It included quite a number of students who had enrolled in the medical course to avoid being drafted. Berg, with his film-star looks, had quite a following. What the class didn't know was that there was a thespian lurking within the heart, if not the mind, of the brilliant molecular chemist.

Members of the class produced a short film - a "molecular feature" featuring costumed dancers wearing body paint and gyrating on a grassy field supposedly representing amino acids, and other bodies within a cell.

Sensing something was afoot, Berg made some discreet enquiries and much to the surprise of the students, joined in enthusiastically – not in the acting or the choreography (!) but by contributing substantially to the funding of the project.

He also approached the team of students who were the producers to "offer his services." Berg wanted to be the invisible narrator and was immediately assigned the role. He tried to disguise his voice but failed miserably as evidenced by his class cheering their popular teacher as soon as he started speaking.

Berg's Final Years.

Berg continued with work in his laboratory at Stanford for 20 years after winning his Nobel prize. He directed research and guided younger researchers from 1985 until his retirement in 2000.

Although he had initially frowned upon the involvement of university professors, including Boyer, with commercial companies, he himself entered the commercial field in 1980, when he became a co-founder of the DNAX biotechnology research Institute, which was later bought by the life sciences company, Schering-

Plough. Researchers from that institute used the technology Berg had developed in his laboratory to produce antibodies and other molecules.

Even during his retirement, Berg continued his association with his department at Stanford. His personality and collegial approach inspired several generation of scientists.

Berg, together with Maxine Singer published several books on genetics for the general reader, as well as a biography of the geneticist George Beadle in *George Beadle:An Uncommon Farmer.*

In 2013 he travelled to England to deliver an eulogy at the funeral of Frederick Sanger who died at the age of 95.

Berg died in 2023 just short of the age of 97.

56

THE MAIN CHARACTERS IN MODERN INSULIN'S DISCOVERY

Most, if not all the young scientists involved in the discovery or development of mammalian and later, modern insulin rose from backgrounds of abject obscurity to adorn the pages of history.

In the story of modern insulin it is impossible to miss the similarities with the narratives of the discovery of the mammalian insulin in Toronto. The majority of researchers who pursued the making of modern insulin were young men and women. Some were graduate students. Even Paul Berg, the leader and senior investigator whose development of *recombinant* technology launched biotechnology into a new sphere of medical and industrial advances, was only in his early 40s.

One aspect of their upbringing, which to the best of my knowledge none of them referred to, was that they were acquainted with adversity. I have mentioned this in the descriptions of the three main characters who are featured in the story of modern insulin.

The story of Paul Berg's parents and the adversities visited upon them in Europe before they migrated to America beggars belief. Stanley Cohen, Herbert Boyer and Robert Swanson were all acquainted with the harsh realities of the poverty of their parents.

However, the "New Age" scientists were also similar in more ways than one. In addition to being "whip smart" they had other interests and priorities of the young men of that age. Thus, Herb Boyer was always quick to remind anyone speaking to him that he took part in every anti-war protest rally held in San Francisco while he was a professor at University of California San Francisco (UCSF). What Boyer did not mention was that he, like many of the others who had headed to the West Coast of the United States, was drawn to it more by its sybaritic attractions than the pursuit of scientific excellence.

Cohen, in addition to being the top graduate in his medical course, played the five-string banjo and ukulele. He also wrote pop songs, one of which made it into the hit parade and was released with the popular baritone Billy Ecksteine as the singer.

Another you will meet later had chosen a particular university to do his degree in science because the area boasted several rock climbing challenges. He remains a mystery until his dramatic entrance in this story at a later stage.

The two most prominent scientists in pioneering modern insulin namely Herb Boyer and Stanley Cohen, now aged 87 and 88 respectively, are retired.

Cohen whose joint experiments with Boyer had pioneered recombinant insulin had left after the completion of the laboratory experiments.

Boyer's contribution to modern insulin is an important chapter in this story.

He was more an outdoors-type and has remained interested in football. He was a lineman in his footballing days. In his later years, Boyer rediscovered his passion for fishing which he pursued in California and later in the Arctic region! There's more to this story as you will discover later.

57

SON OF A RAILWAY WORKER: HERBERT WAYNE BOYER (1936–)

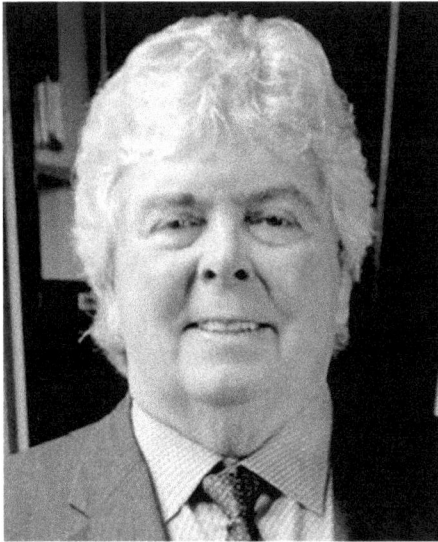

Herbert Wayne Boyer (1936–)

Through direct access to him, Sally Smith Hughes in her book *Genentech* (Chicago University Press 2013) tells of Boyer's humble beginnings from a working class family.

Like Swanson, Boyer had come from a poor family.

Born in 1936, he had grown up on a dairy farm in Pennsylvania. His father and grandfather had worked for the Pennsylvania

Railroad. Young Boyer was very conscious that his father had been forced to leave school at 13 to support his family because his father had died. To support the family, the teenager had worked as a brakeman in the railways.

Boyer never forgot the financial hardships the family endured because his father's limited education had limited his job opportunities to being a brakeman in the railways. Herb was very much an outdoors type, hunting and fishing with his father.

His grades in high school were average. His interests were more in the area of sport and social activities especially football, basketball and baseball. It was his basketball coach, who was also the science and mathematics teacher, who awakened his interest in science and inculcated in the young man the importance of discipline not only in sports but in his studies as well. He later attributed to his football coach a change in his attitude to a more disciplined and consistent approach to studies and later, to life in general. Boyer's grades gradually improved, and he finished high school as the class president while retaining his position in the sporting arena. He played lineman in the football team.

At the age of 23, while still in his first year in graduate school, Boyer married his high school sweetheart, a biology graduate called Marigrace Hensler who at the time was working for a chemical research laboratory. She supported her husband until he completed graduate school.

Boyer gained a bachelor's degree in biology and chemistry in 1958, but did not manage to win a place in medical school.

Although the first in his family to go to college, throughout his life Boyer retained a down-to-earth approach to his dealings with people, and life in general. He eschewed pretentiousness and never forgot his roots nor his working-class upbringing.

In 1954, Boyer went to nearby Saint Vincent College in Latrobe Pennsylvania. There was no family car because his father had never learned to drive, so the college student hitch-hiked or took a bus to his lectures.

Boyer's Lightbulb Moment at College.

It was in college that Boyer developed an interest in chemistry after a particular experience. 50 years after the incident Boyer described it to Sally Smith Hughes.

> *"We had a brand-new shiny cell physiology textbook with a blue and white cover. Each of us was assigned a chapter, and we had to give a seminar on it.*
>
> *This was 1957, and the buzz of DNA was just getting into the textbooks…. I was really taken with the Watson-Crick structure of DNA and this started in my fascination with the heuristic value of the structure."*

Hughes also spoke in her book of Boyer's fascination with the work of the Cambridge scientists which led to his two Siamese cats being named Crick and Watson.

The aspiring chemist and researcher took courses in biology and chemistry.

Fortunately for the easy going Boyer, St. Vincent College was run by Benedictine monks who are known for their insistence on a strict adherence to discipline.

Unfortunately, at the end of college, Boyer's application for admission to medical school was rejected because of his failure in one subject – metaphysics.

Switching to a course in biology at the University of Pittsburgh, Boyer was surprised to find how much he enjoyed bacteriology, especially his time in the laboratory. The interaction with other students who engaged in frequent informal discussions and seminars saw him thrive in his studies

As mentioned above this was the time of the scientific world being awakened to virtually unlimited possibilities following the 1953 discovery of the structure of DNA by the Cambridge duo of Francis Crick and James Watson.

For Boyer in his own words, this "was my awakening."

Just as the discovery of insulin in 1921 by Banting's Toronto team had started "an avalanch" of scientific investigations and experiments into the various aspects of the hormone, so had the double helix of DNA after the Nobel Prize winning discovery by the Cambridge scientists.

Many years later Boyer, commenting on the identification of the three-dimensional structure of DNA by Watson and Crick, said that the finding had

> *"opened the door to many of the advances that were to shape medical and biomedical research for years. The beauty of the structure was evident to just about everyone at the time. The structure presented a very simple way for the chemical (DNA) to explain the fundamentals required for the genetic material to duplicate itself, code for the information that allows our cells to produce all the things necessary for us to be who we are and provide a way for life to evolve."*
>
> (Italics by the author.)

I have quoted Boyer because the explanation he provides for the double helix is an example of his capacity to explain complicated chemistry in simple terms. This is an uncommon gift and an extremely useful one, not only for teachers, but also to explain it to other sections of the community, which in Boyer's case would turn out to be newspaper reporters and later, potential investors. The initial funding for the first biotechnology company was raised after he had explained what biotechnology was to the venture capitalists.

Boyer set himself the ambitious project of deciphering DNA and persisted in spite of the success of the project achieved by the Cambridge scientists in 1961. His supervisor, impressed with Boyer's submission, accepted the dissertation for a doctorate in bacteriology which the university conferred on the popular graduate in 1963.

From Pittsburgh Boyer went to Yale do a post doctoral fellowship in microbiology. It was here that he began his work on the exchange of genetic material in different bacteria. The laboratory he worked in was involved in researching "restriction enzymes." Normally these enzymes destroy any foreign agent which enters the bodies of bacteria.

Boyer continued his studies in bacteria concentrating on the methods for "cutting and pasting" pieces of the twisted ladder of DNA. To do the cutting and pasting the scientists use enzymes. The enzymes which are used for cutting DNA, are called "restriction enzymes".

Remember this was 1963.

Little wonder than that Boyer's expertise in working with DNA would later be of significant assistance to other scientists involved in such work in the early 1970s.

This included a scientist called Paul Berg.

It is important to reflect on comments made by Sally Smith Hughes in her book *Genentech* that even at this early stage of his work on this subject which was to lead to later research in recombinant technology, Boyer gave much thought to the practical uses of the research in which he was engaged,

In 1966 Boyer moved west as an assistant professor in the microbiology department of the University of California, San Francisco (UCSF). Even though the chairman of the department was an "old school" scientist with no interest in molecular genetics, Boyer tolerated the lack of stimulation as well as limited laboratory space in a department which, before his appointment, had promised him space in the university's new research tower. His interest in "the new genetics" to manipulate DNA remained very much to the fore in his thinking.

However, in an interview with Sally Hughes many years later (1975) Boyer said that during the early years in his new appointment he was able to meet and develop friendships with a group of other scientists. He would spend several hours each week discussing with them the pros and cons of genetic engineering as it might affect society.

After four frustrating years, Boyer was still unable to find an enzyme which would cut DNA at a predictable position.

Then fate intervened and as the saying goes, all things come to those who wait.

In 1968 a biochemist, William J. Rutter arrived at UCSF to head the biochemistry department which the university had decided to turn into a premier research institution.

Rutter's approach to improving the department was to broaden the base of research by including different disciplines, and encouraging cooperation between different departments and, what was unusual at that time, between different disciplines.

From Boyer's viewpoint the emphasis on the latest techniques to decipher the genetic make up of higher organisms was very much in alignment with the direction of his own research.

It was exactly what Boyer needed and wanted. He spent longer hours in the biochemistry department, which became his second academic home. The lively seminars, informal discussions, and generally friendly atmosphere suited his outgoing personality.

The biochemistry department – not the bacteriology department which was the location of his official position – became Boyer's second home.

Even at this early stage, Boyer's sixth sense told him that restriction enzymes were important and could play a role in recombining the DNA of bacteria with the DNA of a different organism. However, he had not advanced far enough in this branch of research and studies for the idea to be any more than just that.

His interest in, and fascination with molecular biology which had been awakened in 1957 by his early exposure to studies in the structure of DNA at the hands of his teachers, the Benedictine monks in Saint Vincent College in Latrobe, Pennsylvania where he had enrolled in 1954, had continued unabated. Boyer never forgot his indebtedness to Saint Vincent College, from where he had graduated in 1958 with his Bachelor of Science degree in biology and chemistry.

The Benedictine monks had succeeded in imparting the importance of discipline in the carefree young man who at that time had been more interested in outdoor pursuits, music and girls.

In retirement many years later, Boyer spoke of the teacher who had inspired him. He named the late Fr. Joel Lieb as being instrumental in guiding him in his studies in the formative years.

Some 60 years later, in an interview with Sally Smith Hughes, Boyer could still describe the epiphany (quoted earlier), which had determined the course of his lifelong interest and studies.

As mentioned earlier, in 1966 Boyer had moved to the West Coast of the United States as Assistant Professor of Microbiology at University of California, San Francisco.

Although now a professor, he eschewed every element of elitism often associated with the upper echelons of academia. He wore casual attire – jeans, sneakers, and a leather vest – and depended on his own down-to-earth approach in dealing with colleagues and students alike. Beneath this exterior however, lay a tough and tenacious researcher with an inner dynamism. His capacity for long hours of arduous work in the laboratory was well known to all who worked with him.

One of Boyer's strengths I commented on earlier was his gift of simplifying complicated facts of chemistry and biochemistry especially when explaining them to people outside the academic field.

His lectures to students were popular. More importantly, the same facility permitted him to gain common ground with fellow-researchers in the academic sphere.

Many researchers, though gifted in conducting experiments are not necessarily able to express complicated scientific terms and procedures in the language of the man in the street. Little wonder that Boyer was able to foster a collaborative approach to many related problems which were being pursued in different laboratories and was able to establish partnerships with colleagues and younger scientists for example, post doctoral students. These capabilities were to stand him in good stead in the commercial sector later in his "second" career in the corporate/commercial sphere.

Even as he was working on the commercial side of modern insulin, Boyer had continued with his research on enzymes useful for cutting DNA. and, in academic and research circles, had become well known in his field through his publications and seminars held in San Francisco and further afield during conferences, and through invited lectures.

(In 1989 Boyer and his wife Grace donated $1 million dollars as a gift to the campaign for Saint Vincent College, which created student scholarships in memory of Mrs Boyer's father, T. L. Hensler, and her brother, Timothy. The scholarships have continued and have enabled many students with academic and leadership qualities to attend St Vincent College.)

58

STANLEY NORMAN COHEN (1935 –)
A FATEFUL ASSOCIATION

Like Boyer, Stanley Norman Cohen*, was also the first child in his family. His parents lived in New Jersey, a town a few miles from New York City. Like the Boyers, the Cohens were also a family which struggled with financial hardships.

Like many of the scientists who contributed to the development of modern insulin, Cohen's parents were Jewish immigrants. His father Bernard was an electrician and his mother worked as a secretary and bookkeeper to supplement her husband's earnings. In his childhood, Stanley frequently helped by joining his father at work.

Unlike Herb Boyer, Stan was preternaturally disciplined and intellectually gifted.

Inculcated with religious instruction, he was also a devout follower of his family's Jewish faith to which he adhered with lifelong respect and strict adherence to its norms and mores. He regularly read the Torah and Talmud which he could recite.

Aiming to be a physician, Cohen studied biology. He went to Rutgers University where he graduated top of his class in Medicine in 1960.

Within three years of graduation, in addition to his internship, Cohen completed a residency in medicine and a two-year research position in the National Institutes of Health (NIH).

Determined to achieve work - life balance, Cohen learned to play the guitar and wrote pop-songs one of which was picked up by a recording studio and later released with the popular singer Billy Ecksteine as the vocalist.

A chance meeting in 1972, with Herb Boyer, led to a fruitful collaboration which in 1973 carried out the critical experiments with E.coli bacteria to produce recombinant DNA. Their widely hailed work, the success of which paved the way for the widespread adoption of genetic engineering in research laboratories as well as in industrial settings, is part of the early history of biotechnology. The revolutionary new technologies which Boyer's and Cohen's research helped develop opened hitherto undreamt of possibilities for the production of hormones such as insulin in test tubes without relying on animal pancreases which had been introduced following their use in the discovery of insulin by Banting and Best in 1921.

Once the exercise of producing recombinant insulin had been accomplished, the two scientists returned to separate scientific pursuits in the second half of 1975. Cohen also joined the biotechnology company called Cetus in an advisory capacity while continuing with his academic and research activities. More than once Cohen had said he preferred to conduct his research alone.

After his collaboration with Cohen, Boyer returned to his laboratory and teaching commitments at USFC.

Fortunately for science in general and diabetes in particular fate had conspired to lead Boyer in an entirely unexpected direction.

*(not to be confused with Stanley Cohen, the 1986 Nobel Prize winner in Medicine or Physiology for his work on growth factors).

The number of participants in this exercise required the contributions of far more than the team of four credited with the discovery of insulin in 1921.

It is at this point that the story gets more interesting because we meet some remarkable and colourful individuals. Whether they dispel or confirm some of the myths and stereotypes which are at times associated with "academic types" I shall leave to the reader.

59

THE HONOLULU DELI INCIDENT

"We are pilgrims on a journey,
We are brothers on the road…"
The Servant Song by Richard Gillard, 1977.

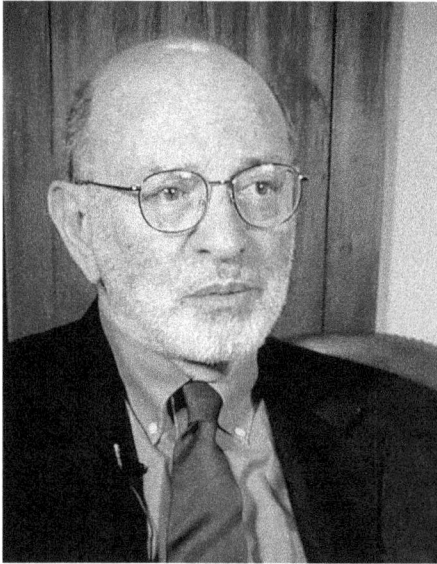

Stanley Norman Cohen (1935–)

Stanley Norman Cohen.
A Brilliant Researcher.

Late 1972 is an important period in the history of new insulin because critical decisions were made by two previously unacquainted scientists. Their names were Herbert Wayne Boyer and Stanley Norman Cohen.

They were young men of the same age and backgrounds but with markedly different outlooks on professional and personal fronts. To meet in a tropical island and collaborate in a critical, early phase of the development of a "new" insulin had not occurred to either of them.

Although both Cohen and Boyer had shared interests through working on related research projects, their personalities were very different. Boyer was gregarious, open and outgoing. He made friends easily.

Cohen on the other hand, was a quiet achiever. He was also a loner. Intense and productive he was inclined to keep to himself, almost to the point of secrecy. Sally Smith Hughes in her book *Genentech* commented that Cohen worked on the principle of the whale which stayed underwater to avoid being harpooned if it raised its head above the waves.

The best account of their initial meeting is an article which Stanley Cohen published in the Proceedings of the National Academy of Sciences.

In November 1972, Boyer travelled to Hawaii for a conference on microbiology. This was the time and place where the "Hatched in a Honolulu Deli" story took place.

At this point in time, which was the summer of 1972, Cohen had come to a roadblock in his own research. He and his team were frustrated in their attempts to join pieces of DNA.

It is unlikely that he would have allowed himself the luxury of speculating that a joint research carried out by him with equally important contributions by Boyer would lead to a veritable explosion in experiments related to biotechnology. That this, in turn would open the way for entrepreneurs and industry to use their methods of working with DNA which had been pioneered in their laboratories had not occurred to either of the two young scientists. There are several versions of the story of Boyer and Cohen's first meeting but this one is largely based on Cohen's own account.

Cohen had heard that a graduate student in Boyer's laboratory had succeeded in an exercise set by Boyer which involved cutting DNA into pieces at specific positions in the molecule.

This was precisely what Cohen had wanted to accomplish but had been frustrated in his attempts to that point in time.

All this had happened at a time when Cohen was in the process of organising a conference on the subject related to his own experiments which he now realised were also closely related to Boyer's research.

The conference was a joint venture between United States and Japan. It had been jointly organised by Cohen together with help from Tsutomu Watanabe, a respected pioneer in the studies of bacterial antibiotic resistance, and Donald Helsinki, a scientist who was also involved in the early stages of recombinant research.

It was Helsinki who having learned of Boyer's work which happened to be directly related to the subjects to be covered in the conference, suggested to Cohen that Boyer be added to the list of speakers. Given that the conference was only a few weeks away, Cohen telephoned Boyer who, being the easygoing individual he was said, "sure."

In my reading on the subject I found an interesting reference to the meeting in Hawaii in a brief article (from the DNA Learning Centre from the Cold Spring Harbour Laboratory).

It said that "… in 1972, at a meeting in Hawaii, Cohen sat in on a talk by Herbert Boyer, who spoke about how a restriction enzyme *EcoRI* generated sticky ends…. and recombinant DNA technology was born on a Deli napkin. Cohen and Boyer eventually patented the technique – one of the first biotech patents granted."

A similar example of the readiness of Herb Boyer to share his findings with colleagues involved Art Riggs, the head of the group of scientists from the City of Hope Laboratories who would later collaborate with Boyer to pioneer the commercial production of recombinant insulin.

By an interesting coincidence Riggs' interest in the possibility of making recombinant insulin had also begun after attending "a seminar given by a young professor from UCSF" the young professor was Herb Boyer.

In both instances Boyer's contributions, which were of critical importance in moving forward the research on recombinant insulin received, at least in my opinion, less publicity and recognition than they deserved. To say that Boyer was unassuming individual would be an understatement.

Cohen and Boyer's Critical Experiment.

"I looked at the first gels, and I remember tears coming into my eyes, it was so nice."

Herb Boyer's reaction on seeing the first gels of Boyer - Cohen recombinant molecules.

The story of the Boyer-Cohen collaboration began on the evening of the first day of the conference. The group had had a meal provided at the venue of the meetings. The dinner, typical of dinners in scientific conferences, had been of average quality and quantity. Neither Cohen nor Boyer had had enough to eat.

According to Cohen, "the actual collaboration began during a long walk near Honolulu's Waikiki beach in search of a sandwich shop to have a late evening snack."

The group also included the popular bacteriologist Stanley Falcow.

They stopped at a quiet, dark street near Waikiki Beach when they came across a New York-style deli which unlike most shops, had the window sign of welcome which read "Shalom" instead of, as the devout Cohen put it, "the ubiquitous Aloha."

While strolling on Waikiki Beach earlier, Cohen and Boyer had described their respective experiments to each other which, at that time, neither had published.

By that time they came across the deli, they had already decided to collaborate and had agreed on the basic plan for the joint project. As recalled by Cohen,

"A few minutes later, over warm pastrami and corned beef sandwich and cold beer, Herb and I sketched out an experimental plan on napkins taken from the dispenser at our table."

The framed cartoon-like drawing of that conference in the deli is part of the history of Waikiki Beach. It was published in the Honolulu Advertiser newspaper on September 26, 1988. The paper reported that the "Waikiki beach delicatessen, where the initial DNA cloning experiments were planned" was to be demolished.

It was during this discussion, that both Cohen and Boyer realised how bacteria could be harnessed to produce modern "recombinant" insulin.

Remember, it was Boyer who had helped Berg's assistant Janet Mertz overcome an early problem.

Here, once again, Boyer saw the potential benefits in combining the method he had developed with laboratory techniques which were being used by Cohen.

And once again, as he had done with Berg's work, Boyer was prepared to supply the material he had developed to Cohen. However Cohen insisted that the work be done through a collaboration between the two. Commenting on this many years later through oral history recorded in 2009 and quoted by Sally Smith Hughes in her book *Genentech,* Cohen, when offered the material which Boyer had developed had said,

"Well, that doesn't seem quite fair. Your lab has spent a lot of time isolating the enzyme, and we should do this as a collaboration."

What Cohen also realised was that Boyer, beneath his bluff easy-going exterior was in fact, blessed with a razor-sharp intellect, and a capacity for working long hours in the laboratory. Another characteristic of Boyer's character was to underplay his expertise in, and knowledge of, ways of working with the enzymes needed for cutting pieces of DNA.

Then followed a period of frantic activity and cooperation between the two laboratories with material being ferried from one to the other in the car (a Volkswagen "beetle") owned by one of one of Cohen's research associates.

A new member of the team assembled by Cohen and Boyer was John Morrow, a graduate student of Paul Berg. For the experiment the team had in mind they needed an animal DNA to combine with the bacterial material. Morrow told Boyer that he had a sample of DNA from a frog which had been prepared by one of his mentors. Morrow checked with his mentor who, as was common in the research community, was generous and willing to provide the sample for Boyer's experiment.

In July 1973, the Cohen-Boyer team succeeded in joining the genetic material from two different and unrelated organisms, namely a frog and a bacterium, to create a single new "recombinant" entity.

(The actual date of the experiment is unclear. July, 1973 is the date mentioned in Sally Smith Hughes' *Genentech*. In Mukherjee's *The Gene* it was on New Year's Day 1974 that "a researcher working with Cohen at Stanford reported reported that he had inserted a frog gene into a bacterial cell."

In essence, the exercise can be described as follows:

When a minute number, such as a single colony of bacteria, containing the frog gene, had been injected in a quantity of sterile bacterial broth, overnight the single colony had made copies of itself and produced over 1 million copies of an entirely new organism.

A new life had been created by combining two unrelated organisms in a test tube.

Boyer was beside himself.

A colleague, having heard the news and considering it extremely unlikely, telephoned Boyer. Being familiar with the frog prince fable, the gregarious scientist could not help himself.

As described in Hughes' book *Genentech,*

"Herb," the colleague reported, "just said he kissed every bacterial colony on the culture plate until one turned into a prince. Then he hung up, and I had to call again to get the real answer."

Modern insulin searched for, sought after, and pursued for thousands of years had emerged, no, catapulted out of a glass test tube in a research laboratory in San Francisco in July 1973.

Berg's recombinant technology had enabled Boyer and Cohen to discovered Cinderella's glass slipper.

The significance of this is hard to overstate.

Boyer realised this and never forgot it.

Just as John Jacob Abel had described the moment in 1926 when he saw insulin crystals as "the most beautiful sight," Boyer's reaction in his own words was quoted by Mukherjee:

"I looked at the first gels, and I remember tears coming into my eyes, it was so nice."

For Cohen that it was *"elation."*

Mukherjee, a medical graduate, also couldn't help himself, saying this was "as close to metaphysics as one can get." He was probably referring to the low marks Boyer had scored in the one subject which had prevented him from gaining entry into medical school.

That subject was metaphysics.

The medical profession's loss was medical research's gain and millions of men, women and children who use insulin every day were the benefactors – as were the millions of animals whose lives were spared.

In May1974 Cohen published a paper describing the successful transfer of a frog gene into a bacterial cell.

(As noted above, for the purposes of this account the exact date of publication is probably not of crucial importance but according to Mukherjee a researcher working with Cohen at Stanford had reported on New Year's Day 1974 that he had inserted a frog gene into a bacterial cell).

The critical importance of this achievement was the combination of two very different "organisms" on the evolutionary ladder, the frog, being a more "advanced" form of life compared to bacteria.

60

THE END OF AN HISTORIC COLLABORATION

The Boyer and Cohen partnership, although brief in terms of the time the two scientists spent together, made a critical contribution to the biotechnology which eventually led to making modern insulin. They pioneered a method of cloning genetically engineered molecules in foreign cells. The application of this discovery was an important early breakthrough in the lead up to today's biotechnology industry.

The revolutionary technique opened hitherto unimagined, and unimaginable, possibilities for the role of genes in many biological, industrial, agricultural and pharmaceutical fields.

The enormous possibilities suggested by Boyer's and Cohen's experiments did not escape the notice of the scientific community.

Mukherjee, who was a student in Berg's laboratory in 1993, described this in his usual inimitable fashion:

> *Recombinant DNA had pushed genetics from the realm of science into the realm of technology. Genes were not abstractions any more. They could be liberated from the genomes of organisms, where they had been trapped for millenia, shuffled between species, amplified, purified, extended, shortened, altered, remixed, mutated, mixed, matched, cut, pasted, edited; they were infinitely malleable to human intervention. Genes were no longer just the subjects of study, but the instrument of study."*

(Italics by author).

It was the use of genes as an instrument of study which was to culminate in the production of modern insulin.

The potential of this was hard to miss.

Stanford put out "a news flash" and quoted Joshua Lederberg, a Nobel Laureate's speculation that the experiment might "completely change the pharmaceutical industry's approach to making biological elements, such as <u>insulin</u> and antibiotics."

(underline by author).

Even now, some 50 years after the creation of the first recombinant molecule, there is still only partial awareness (and understanding) of the processes, now proven, and their potential for advances in the understanding of the nature of genes even though genetic engineering is now widely used in the laboratories of scientists working on products ranging from pharmaceutical to agricultural formulations.

Inherent weaknesses previously regarded as incurable, could now be eliminated by newly-developed technologies. Changes believed to have evolved over some billions of years could, with the new technologies, be altered, improved or eliminated.

As Cohen himself observed, scientists could now intervene in conditions which had existed over two billions years in what we called – and still call – evolution.

Nature was no longer unchangeable and absolute. Genes in humans which were previously considered sacrosanct were now being sliced, diced and tossed around.

If this wasn't science-fiction come to life, I don't know what is.

In spite of the spectacular results of the collaboration which occupies a unique place in medical history, the publication of the experiments by Boyer and Cohen marked the end of the partnership between the two brilliant young men.

The two "brothers in science", whose collaborative experience and experiments will remain a part of history, ended their journey in 1974, less than two years after their discussion in the delicatessen on Waikiki Beach in Honolulu.

In 1974 Boyer and Cohen parted company to pursue their individual goals. Boyer returned to his academic position, and Cohen to his own research. Cohen had also secured an advisory position on the board of a biotechnology company.

How Did the Boyer and Cohen Research Relate to Asilomar ?

Neither Cohen nor Boyer had any doubts about the need to press on with the research on recombinant technology to produce recombinant insulin through the technique which has been discovered by Berg only recently. They had continued with experiments during and after the period of the Asilimar conferences.

That they were both aware of the issues to be addressed in the conference is supported by the letters from Cohen to Paul Berg.

Copies of these are preserved in the Paul Berg Papers in the National Library of Medicine.

For the two scientists, Cohen and Boyer, this was a very difficult period. The machinations of internal politics especially in academic circles produced open disagreement, conflict and hostility.

Even years later, as recorded in the oral history archives quoted by Sally Smith Hughes, Boyer recalled the sense of isolation he experienced when criticised by those he had considered friends within the academic circles in which he had worked, and thrived, for many years.

One of his colleagues referred to this period as "a harrowing time for Herb Boyer."

Boyer himself admitted to being confused by the reactions of some of his colleagues saying, "Here I thought I was doing something that was valuable to society, and doing something that would make a contribution, and then to have the accusations and criticisms, it was extremely difficult."

Neither he nor Cohen considered the Asilomar meetings helpful to the project of developing genetic engineering for biological purposes. Contrary to some reports including at least one article online, Cohen refused to sign the preliminary draft of the guidelines for recombinant research. Boyer called the conference "a nightmare."

The experiment conducted by Boyer and Cohen, which made critical contributions to the development of genetic engineering by employing recombinant technology was published in several scientific papers.

As mentioned earlier, it also marked the end of their collaboration in 1974. Boyer returned to his microbiology laboratory at the University of California to continue his research believing that beyond the publication of his and Cohen's findings in scientific journals, their work, like many scientific studies and research, was not likely to go any further. How wrong he was!

61

A 3- HR. PUB LUNCH IN A SAN FRANCISCO COCKTAIL BAR

One drink led to another…

It is not part of my brief to create controversy, but some may consider my next statement provocative or one which at least invites questions if not speculations.

Genentech, the first commercial enterprise, which produced modern recombinant insulin for the use of patients would not have been created were it not for the drive and enthusiasm of a young man who was an outsider in this company of academically accomplished and often "driven" scientists.

His name was Robert Swanson.

Swanson had no claim to academic distinction, but he was certainly driven.

So what is the Robert Swanson story?

Was he a distinguished scholar?

A respected researcher?

A famous professor?

A Nobel Laureate?

The answer is, "None of the above."

If nothing else, the choice should reassure and encourage us mere mortals, because the man who I believe was most responsible for the critical step of bringing insulin out of the laboratory to the men, women and children with diabetes was not a doctor, nor even a scientist.

He was a "people person."

His name was Bob Swanson.

Little did Boyer know that after the end of his collaboration with Cohen when he believed that fate had relegated him to the backwaters of research, his career would take off on a steep upward trajectory. Perhaps the gods had not forgotten the sacrifices made by Boyer's father, a 13-year-old who had given up school and worked as a shift worker for Pennsylvania Railways to support the family. Although he made time to engage in outdoor activities such as fishing with his son, the father had always impressed on young Herb the importance of hard, honest labour.

In January 1976 Boyer took a phone call from a stranger called Robert Swanson asking to meet him for a brief meeting to discuss the commercial possibilities of the recombinant technique. Like most medical graduates, Boyer was entirely unversed in matters commercial and like most individuals who have been acquainted with poverty especially in their formative years, his memories of deprivation due to financial hardship had not been forgotten.

Boyer agreed to the proposed meeting in a pub but told Swanson that he could only spare a few minutes.

In an interview many years later, Boyer recalled his initial meeting with Swanson. He thought, but was not entirely certain, that he had agreed to meet Bob Swanson in a local cocktail bar called Churchill's which was located on Clement Street in the shopping precinct of the city. Swanson's enthusiasm coupled with an infectious friendliness impressed Boyer, who was more than 10 years older.

What impressed the academic researcher even more was that although the idea of making drugs in the laboratory had occurred to him previously, it had not borne fruit because a chemist whom Boyer had supplied with the necessary materials, although interested at first, had not been able to produce a marketable product as he had promised.

The "few minutes" stretched into a three-hour meeting between Boyer and the aspiring entrepreneur largely because whatever problems and questions troubled the scientist, Swanson was a jump ahead not only because he had faced them himself, but more importantly, had constructive suggestions for ways to overcome them.

"What about the money"? Boyer had asked.

"Venture capitalists," was the answer.

It is possible that Boyer might not have known the meaning of the term let alone the basics of raising capital. The commercial aspects were far removed from the knowledge and expertise of the scientists including the leaders and professors in the research community within the academic settings of university departments.

The pair quickly recognised each other's complementary capabilities, namely Boyer's scientific expertise and Swanson's knowledge of creating and financing a commercial company.

They also recognised that they both shared a vision, and a down-to earth-approach to challenges.

What neither of them, to the best of my knowledge, ever mentioned was that both had memories and experience of poverty. Swanson had tasted hard times more recently including at the time of his meeting with Boyer. He would never forget that at the time he was living on unemployment benefits.

In spite of their compatibility, it is entirely possible that had Boyer known about Swanson's background, including his recent failed foray into venture capitalism, the affable academic may have had second thoughts about entering into the partnership.

62

THE UNSUNG HERO OF
MODERN INSULIN

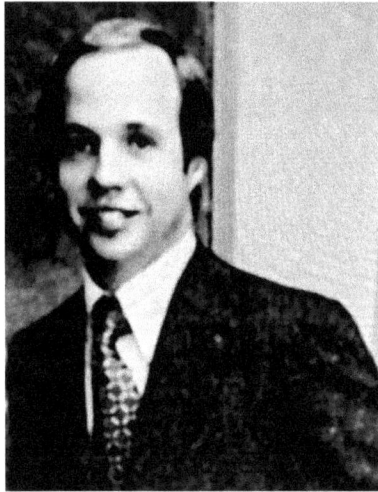

Robert Arthur Swanson.

Robert Swanson (1947–1999).

The new recombinant insulin was produced through the cooperative and coordinated efforts of many individuals – many, because each step was so complicated that it required the combined contributions of several scientists each with his/her own expertise in a particular area - to the stage of identifying and complying with the legal requirements of patenting, registering and financing the project. The legal steps for application to various statutory bodies as well the

the commercial aspects were far removed from the knowledge and expertise of the scientists including the leaders and professors in the research community.

It is also an appropriate time to emphasise that each one of these men led a group of associates in several related but highly specialised areas of research involving recombinant insulin.

For the majority of such scientists, the commercial aspect of their lives is restricted to their salary. The world of owning shares in a commercially viable enterprise which was being planned by Swanson was entirely outside the mindset of men like Boyer as well as the scientists who were to join him later. This was noted by David Goeddel in an interview some years after he had experienced the corporate world.

Robert Arthur Swanson (1947–1999), was a Brooklyn–born, only child of a family of humble means whose father was the head of an airline maintenance crew in Miami. An aptitude in mathematics and science led to Swanson's entry to the prestigious Massachusetts Institute of technology (MIT) in 1965. The 18-year-old enjoyed the camaraderie in the institution and realised that he was a "people person". Sally Smith Hughes in her book *Genentech* (Chicago University Press 2011) spoke of Swanson being "a doer, not a thinker."

One decision during his time at MIT had a more profound effect than has been acknowledged. On his own initiative, Swanson made a decision to interrupt his MIT course and enrol in the Sloan School of Management. The curriculum in the business school included studies of entrepreneurship which includes the development of organisational skills. At that time Venture capitalists were in their infancy. Swanson learnt the basics of preparing business plans. He was excited by the prospect of ideas leading to practical results, such as a new product associated with or leading to starting new business enterprises. Suffice it to say that in 1970, the 23 year-old graduated from MIT with not only a Bachelors degree in Chemistry but also a Masters in Management.

An early contact with venture capitalists Eugene Kleiner and Thomas Perkins, who had founded Kleiner and Perkins in 1972, led to the ambitious entrepreneur's first job as a junior partner.with the firm in late 1974. Importantly, this was to be Swanson's first contact with a company contemplating the use of an emerging technology called recombinant DNA because Kleiner and Perkins had invested in a company called Cetus Corporation.

(The company had acquired the name Cetus when one of its senior founders, while swimming, had been bitten by what he thought was a whale but which was later found to be a small shark. However, the decision was made to stick with the original name Cetus which is latin for whale).

Kleiner and Perkins became concerned with the lack of progress in Cetus and assigned to Swanson the task of monitoring the firm's progress and also to look into its investment procedures.

In 1975 Swanson arranged a lunch with Cetus executives and cofounders, including the Nobel laureate Donald Glaser, Peter Farley, and Ron Cape. (Donald Glaser's Nobel Prize in 1960 was for Physics)

Peter Farley (1940 – 2010), was also familiar with the technology because he had a background in medicine, having been a medical officer in a nuclear submarine. He was also the first physician to enrol at Harvard University for a course on business studies which had led to an MBA. He was the one who had been bitten by a shark - not a whale.

Unfortunately, the attempt by Swanson and Perkins to fire up the company, including the use of emerging technologies – recombinant DNA was mentioned – had little effect.

(Stanley Cohen, later a leading authority on the revolutionary recombinant technology, was not to join Cetus till some years later).

In spite of the potential for financial profits which had been trumpeted by the exuberant Bob Swanson, the meeting failed to get any meaningful response from the Cetus team. Shortly afterwards Kleiner and Perkins terminated their relationship with the company and, unfortunately for Swanson, advised him that they could no longer needed his services.

The luncheon however, had one significant outcome. Donald Glaser, who was a friend of Cohen, had emphasised the possibilities of genetic engineering and, without explaining how, the potential of significant financial returns from its use.

Unlike the other men at the luncheon, Glaser had found a convert in young Bob Swanson who had already seen see a definite potential for the use of the new technology to make significant profits.

At that time however, Swanson being unemployed and living off the benefits cheque of around $400 a month, could do little about it.

Yet even though his impecunious state forced him to explore many options – anything to pay his rent – Swanson kept thinking about recombinant DNA and the potential of the revolutionary technology for making money.

The vision was becoming a driving force.

He had also come to another realisation, which was that raising capital for other commercial firms was, as he put it, "like being a coach on the sidelines."

He decided that he wanted to make money through his own company, not as an employee of another business concern.

63

THE GENENTECH STORY

The Story of a Pioneering Biotechnology Company.

Life must be lived as play.

Plato.

People rarely succeed, unless they have fun in what they are doing.

Andrew Carnegie.

Big Money in Small Molecules.

Swanson had only heard of the new technology based on Paul Berg's revolutionary discovery. He had also managed to find a publicity brochure which listed the participants in a conference on recombinant technology which had been held in Asilomar, a town situated on the Pacific Coast in California. He had no idea what the word recombinant meant. Then again, few people at that time would have known the meaning of a word which had been fashioned by a molecular chemist only a few years earlier.

The participants listed in the brochure were all scientists and Swanson had not heard of a single one of them. Not that this was going to deter the eager and ambitious – but unemployed – entrepreneur.

It is also unlikely that he would have even heard of recombinant technology let alone what it meant, except that his sixth sense told him of its commercial possibilities.

Robert Swanson saw the potential of biotechnology as a player in the high-stakes financial industry and was prepared to back his hunch.

"Big money in small molecules" was more a "gut feeling" for him.

However, he had two problems. He knew nothing about biotechnology and he had empty pockets.

What he did know was that he needed to find a scientist who had been involved in the recombinant DNA project, and with whom he could discuss the project he had in mind.

Swanson decided to cold-call the participants. Most did not return his calls and a few who did gave him short shrift. Fortune favours the brave is a cliche but one which certainly applied to Swanson's search for a scientist?

Eventually he managed a brief conversation with a scientist. That scientist happened to be a professor called Herb Boyer.

Swanson could not possibly have known how fortunate he was to meet Boyer. He certainly did not have the information on, or knowledge of, Boyer's standing within the scientific community or of his expertise in the emerging field of recombinant technology.

Just how fortunate the aspiring, but unemployed, venture capitalist was to have found Boyer would be seen repeatedly in their association for the rest of Swanson's life.

As it turned out, with the contribution of Boyer's expertise in recombinant technology, Robert Swanson played a pivotal role in the modern journey of insulin from its development to the point of making it available as a pharmaceutical product for the use of men, women, and children with diabetes.

It is unclear whether Swanson knew of the prevailing attitude within the scientific community of the feasibility of recombinant technology as a commercial instrument. Although many agreed with its commercial potential, the transition from the laboratory to the manufacturing plants was, in their view, some years away. For example Ron Cape, one of the founders of Cetus Corporation stated that the time frame for the technology to reach profitable commercial levels would require around 10 years. Given that this was said in 1978, provides an indication of the difference between the perceptions of the scientific and the business communities. The former, being extremely cautious, needed all the bases covered before proceeding. Entrepreneurs, like venture capitalists, are not known for patience when it comes to making a profit. They want to feel certain about the chances of a commercial project being successful, (read making money), before risking their capital.

Academia and Pragmatism. The Harsh Realities.

In some ways Swanson's contribution to the story of modern insulin is a combination of the parts played by Banting and Clowes. Remember that Clowse had walked back to the hotel with Macleod after the first public report of Banting and Best's discovery in the annual meeting of the American Physiological Society in New Haven on 20 December 1921. As Lilly's Sales Director he was keen to establish a partnership with the academic and the highest placed "official," Macleod.

Later Clowes and Josiah Lilly, the head of the pharmaceutical company had helped the inexperienced researchers to overcome the many hurdles to eventually produce insulin of an acceptable standard and in sufficient quantities for the use of patients with diabetes.

A similar pattern emerged at this point in the story of modern insulin.

It was the single-mindedness and an uncompromising attitude best demonstrated in the role played by Bob Swanson which, through the cooperation, contributions and drive of a team of researchers and scientists who were also motivated and determined to develop the new product to the point of manufacturing and then marketing it to the public, that insulin was made available to the patients with diabetes.

Some may see an irony in the plan which eventually led to the production of modern insulin being born in the mind of an individual who was neither a scientist nor a research chemist. Rather, it was the result of a desperate attempt by a young man to use a recently discovered and revolutionary biological technique to lift him out of poverty.

As it turned out, Robert Swanson played a pivotal role in the modern journey of insulin. Like Banting, Swanson took synthetic insulin after its discovery to the point of making it available as the treatment for diabetes.

Within months of launching the fledgling commercial company Genentech, Swanson had established a licensed arrangement for Lilly – yes, the same company which had helped launch insulin following its discovery in Toronto – to market modern insulin produced by Genentech.

Thus there are striking similarities between the final, critical steps of delivering insulin to patients with diabetes in the two discoveries of the hormone, namely insulin from animals discovered in Toronto in 1921, and it's synthesis in a test tube in San Francisco in 1978.

Returning to the beginning of the story of Swanson's effort to raise money for Genentech, it is now part of modern insulin's history that capital was eventually raised through Kleiner and Perkins, the same firm for which Swanson had worked previously and from which he had been sacked. The financiers were persuaded not by Swanson's enthusiasm but by the succinct and clear explanation of the method of making recombinant insulin as explained by Boyer.

So Boyer the scientist, together with Robert Swanson, the venture capitalist, founded the first biotechnology company called *Genentech,* a contraction of *gen*etic, *en*gineering, and *tech*nology, thought up by Boyer.

Genentech was the first biotechnology firm to market a pharmaceutical product for human use. It occupies a unique position in history as the first pharmaceutical concern which commercialised recombinant DNA technology to produce insulin in marketable quantities.

Swanson was the company President and Boyer, its Vice President from 1976 to 1991.

Swanson hired premises in a warehouse in San Francisco.

Boyer was the only scientist in the company, which started off with two employees, the other being Swanson.

Late in 1977 Boyer and Swanson hired Dennis Kleid an organic chemist trained in DNA synthesis and molecular biology. They were somewhat taken aback when Kleid said that he would not join Genentech unless his junior associate David Goeddel was was also hired. Goeddel was Kleid's junior colleague at Stanford Research Institute. The strapping young graduate aged 26 years, was a passionate rock-climber and harboured none of Kleid's doubts about joining a newly established firm, which Genentech was. Goeddel started at Genentech in mid-March 1978, and Kleid joined a month later in April.

Genentech's third scientist was the 26-year-old Daniel Yansura, a former University of Colorado lab partner of Goeddel's.

Late in 1977, Irving Johnson, a Lilly employee heard of Genentech more through Swanson's enthusiasm than any documented previous success of the company in products of molecular biology, persuaded his superiors to enter into a contract to help fund research on synthetic insulin at $50,000 per month. At the same time the cautious and experienced Lilly operatives had entered into a similar agreement for the same project with the University of California the previous March.

Also in its very first year of operations, Genentech, through Swanson, contracted to engage researchers at the City of Hope National Medical Centre located outside Los Angeles. The stated aim of the new alliance was to pursue the synthesis of a human gene to produce insulin. The chief scientist of the City of Hope team was Arthur "Art" Riggs (1940 2022), and the molecular biologist was Keiichi Itakura.

Eventually, the team of Boyer, Kleid and Goeddel, when combined with the City of Hope researchers numbered eleven scientists.

Genentech's focus, was to use a recently developed technology, which used bacteria which had been genetically changed for mass production of human proteins, such as insulin and growth hormone and which could then be used for treating the appropriate disorders associated with the lack of these hormones in patients with diabetes and individuals with stunted growth respectively.

64

A THREE – HORSE RACE WON BY THE UNDERDOG!

An unlikely winner is always a good subject for the written and spoken accounts of defeating opponents considered "superior," be it through reputation, size, wealth or prestige. When the story contains all these elements, it becomes an irresistible subject.

The two most important steps in the development of modern insulin were the discovery of genetic engineering, and secondly, the application of this technology to produce the hormone.

The seminal contribution which led to the discovery of recombinant technology by Paul Berg has been related earlier.

However what is often not stated, possibly because it is obvious, is that the scientific breakthrough, significant and dramatic as it was, would not have benefited the millions of patients with diabetes unless modern insulin could be produced on an industrial scale by pharmaceutical companies with established and practical practices of marketing as well as ensuring a continuity of supply. Such activities were well beyond the experience and expertise of research scientists who, as academics, were usually inexperienced in the commercial realities of retail and wholesale pharmacy.

To tell the story of the pursuit of recombinant insulin by using Berg's method of genetic engineering I have chosen the three teams of scientists in America who were researching ways to produce recombinant insulin. Other teams of researchers were also working on the same projects. This included a team in Toronto where insulin had been discovered by Banting and his team.

Stephen Hall in his book, *Invisible Frontiers: The Race to Synthesise a Human Gene* (Sidgwick and Jackson 1988) characterises the efforts of the three groups of scientists as a "race" to be the first to produce synthetic insulin using the recombinant technique.

A similar description was used by Mukherjee when describing the contest between the three teams in his book *The Gene* (Scribner 2016). The prestigious university-based teams at Harvard and UCSF when pitched against the small, newly established biotechnology company Genentech was likened to a David and Goliath contest.

More importantly, for the young chemists working for Genentech especially Goeddel and Yansura the project of making synthetic insulin was very much a contest, as much with the project, as with the other teams of the prestigious university groups of Harvard and UCSF.

Even though I have used a racing analogy in the title, I believe a more productive approach to this part of the modern insulin story would be to look at the three teams through their overall strategies and the emphasis each gave to the specific challenge of making synthetic insulin by using recombinant technology.

The team from Harvard University was led by Walter Gilbert (1932–), a physicist by training and a highly respected scientist with a faultless pedigree in research.

Gilbert had become interested in molecular biology through an acquaintance with James Watson of the double helix fame when Gilbert's wife was working for Watson. Gilbert's work included his Nobel prize-winning contribution to a method of sequencing DNA, which was different from the method pioneered by Frederick Sanger. Both were awarded the Nobel Prize for Chemistry in 1980. (Each received 25% of the monetary award while 50% of the prize was awarded to Paul Berg.)

As far as research on insulin was concerned, Gilbert's laboratory treated that as one of several projects which were being pursued at that time.

However, it must be noted that Gilbert himself took charge of pursuing the synthesis of insulin.

Secondly, William Rutter and Howard Goodman, both from UCSF decided to collaborate on insulin research in order to produce recombinant insulin. Rutter was the Professor of Biochemistry and President of the Chiron Corporation.

Howard Goodman had previously worked with Herb Boyer and had brought his experience in recombinant technology which was greater than that of any other scientist in Rutter's laboratory.

Rutter himself had pursued a more general experimental goal on the pancreas, rather than specifically on insulin. like the Harvard team, the UCSF was also hamstrung by similar governmental restrictions. Rutter's team also included the brilliant Australian cloner, John Shine.

The third team almost didn't "make the cut" to be included in the story.

Herbert Boyer who after the end of his collaboration with Stan Cohen had returned to his previous position of Professor of Microbiology at USCF worked out of a laboratory which was smaller than those of the two universities mentioned above. He devoted his energy to the construction of the material in cells called vectors. Vectors are DNA molecules which can carry a piece of DNA into another cell. Vectors are especially useful for producing recombinant material.

It was actually a small to medium sized laboratory situated within UCSF. But don't be fooled by the size. By now you, like me, may have changed your opinion of the easy-going, friendly and generous Herb Boyer. beneath the easy-going, friendly exterior was a personality with a steely determination and an enviable capacity for working in the laboratory for long hours, frequently throughout the night.

Boyer, operating out of his laboratory with only one "strength" was in sharp contrast, with the programs being pursued by the University laboratories at Harvard and UCSF described above.

The second point of difference was that unlike the two larger university research teams, Boyer and Swanson were operating through a newly formed and recently registered commercial company called *Genentech*. The story of the company is also part of this drama.

How and why the pursuit played out the way it did has invited comment, questions and controversies ever since.

In December 1976, City of Hope scientists Art Riggs and Keiichi Itakura joined Boyer's lab. through a contract secured by Swanson to explore the making of a human gene with the ultimate aim of producing modern insulin.

Riggs' interest in recombinant insulin had been kindled when he had attended a seminar on the subject held at the City of Hope in 1975. The scientist who had lectured on the subject was none other than Herbert Boyer.

It is difficult to not notice the repeated presence of Boyer at critical points in the story of modern insulin. In summary, in the very early parts of Berg's work, it will be recalled that the tedious process which Berg had called "a biochemists nightmare" had been shortened from six steps to two through the generosity of Boyer, who had supplied an enzyme he had developed to Berg's assistant Janet Metz.

Boyer, the Banting of Modern Insulin.

What has not been given sufficient emphasis in the writings on the subject is the presence of one individual in the scientific as well as the commercial aspects of the modern insulin story.

Boyer's role is the closest to the part played by Banting in the discovery of insulin in 1921. Boyer was the one who was there from the beginning through to the point of delivering modern insulin to those who needed it most – the men, women, and children with diabetes.

After the assistance he had provided to Paul Berg as mentioned above, he had been "discovered" by Stan Cohen as someone who had the very enzyme Cohen needed and the absence of which had virtually stopped Cohen's research. Once again, Boyer was not offended by being invited at the last minute – by phone – to the conference where the way the two to proceed had been planned in the Honolulu deli.

Although the Cohen-Boyer collaboration had ended, their work had opened up the possibility of further experiments which would eventually lead to the development of synthetic insulin. However, at this point at least in the USA, the work had been essentially stopped by the self-imposed moratorium following the Asilomar conference.

After the experiments conducted in conjunction with Boyer following their meeting in Hawaii, Cohen had left to pursue his research projects on his own.

Bob Swanson had appeared on the scene after Cohen's departure. Remember that Boyer was the only scientist to respond to Swanson's request for a meeting which had led to the three-hour session in a San Francisco bar where, among other issues, the idea of forming a commercial company had been explored.

Following the formation of Genentech Boyer's gift of being able to reach individuals and groups unfamiliar with the complicated biochemistry underlying the making of modern insulin had once again come to the fore when the group of newsmen had gathered for the announcement of the launching of Genentech on the stock exchange on the back of modern insulin.

Only Boyer stayed the course. It is for this reason that Herb Boyer occupies a unique place in the account of modern insulin.

Will Boyer be remembered when the second centenary of the discovery of insulin is celebrated as Banting was at the first Centenary in 2021?

The First Test for the New Company.

"I don't want to hear that word, impossible... tell me what you need to get it done."

Robert Swanson to Genentech scientist
Dennis Kleid.

If the two Bs of the Toronto team were Banting and Best, the two men responsible for modern insulin were Berg and Boyer.

The alliterative combinations are little more than perhaps a Trivial Pursuit question.

In both teams one scientist was awarded the Nobel Prize, the other wasn't.

Yet each one deservedly occupies a place of unique distinction in history.

Just as the discovery of insulin had lead to an avalanche of experiments on the hormone, so was the response of the research community to Berg's success in creating a recombinant entity.

As mentioned above the early part of the story of modern insulin includes the story of three different teams of highly qualified and talented scientists with an expertise in molecular chemistry engaging in researching ways to produce recombinant insulin pioneered by Paul Berg.

In addition to the stories mentioned above, *Genentech* by Sally Smith Hughes (published by the University of Chicago Press in 2013), also provides a detailed and interesting account of the competition to produce recombinant insulin.

Another detailed account, replete with technical details, can be found in a National Library of Medicine (NIH) publication written by Scott Stern in 1995.

The single factor, which influenced the outcome of the results achieved by the three teams was Asilomar. The constraints placed on recombinant research proved a stumbling block for the bigger contestants led by Gilbert and Rutter because both were constrained by guidelines which had to be followed by institutions supported by government funds.

To get past the US government's two year moratorium imposed on recombinant research following Asilomar, Gilbert made arrangements with a military establishment in England to continue experiments aimed at producing recombinant insulin.

An additional stumbling block for the Harvard team had arisen from the vigorous, almost belligerent, opposition to any recombinant research being carried out in the Harvard laboratories which were situated in Cambridge, Massachusetts. The mayor of Cambridge, Alfred Velluchi had little time for the prestigious institution generally, and perhaps professors and "white coat merchants" specifically. He made all sorts of threats-and succeeded.

Walter Gilbert decided against engaging in a no-holds-barred public brawl with the combative, wily and experienced politician. Perhaps the letter from Paul Berg to Velluchi as quoted in this book was Berg's way of providing some support to his academic colleague.

Both the "academic" teams attempted the same strategy to get around the problem. Like the Harvard team, the UCSF group sent one of their scientists to a secure laboratory in France.

Unfortunately for both these teams, their failure to produce recombinant insulin was found to be related directly to the decision to move overseas. In each instance, during transport somehow, some of the chemicals had become contaminated and therefore could not be used in the experiments.

Genentech had found a way to get around the funding problem because they did not depend on government support but had used venture capitalists. Neither did they have to move to new facilities. The company conducted the experiments in its usual premises namely, a rented warehouse in San Francisco.

Herb Boyer at University of San Francisco, California (USFC), together with Robert Swanson had formed a team with Arthur Riggs and Keiichi Itakura at the City of Hope National Medical Centre.

Additional team members were drawn from graduate students and postgraduate researchers similar to the team which had worked with Paul Berg. The eventual group included scientists from various parts of the world, including Europe, South America and Australia. in addition to Boyer, Genentech had three more scientists namely Dennis Kleid, Dave Goeddel and Daniel Yansura.

At that time, a senior scientist, Rachmiel Levine (1910–1998) was the Executive Medical Director of the City of Hope. Highly regarded by scientists because of his background in investigating insulin activity but also because of his wisdom and wide range of contacts, Levine encouraged Riggs and Itakura to work with Boyer to develop modern insulin. Riggs repeatedly acknowledged the important role played by the senior scientist.

Such groups were necessary owing to the specialised nature of the projects which needed special skills such as expertise and experience in the use of particular instruments. The leaders of the teams, by virtue of age and experience, were more the go–to individuals who also attended to administrative needs and provided guidance for the younger members of each team. The senior members of a department were often experienced researchers themselves.

Yet, in spite of having a formidable team of researchers, Boyer hesitated. Why?

The reason was the same as that which had stayed the hand of Dorothy Hodgkin in Bernal's laboratory in Oxford University decades earlier.

It was the daunting size of the insulin molecule.

Mukherjee, who hails from Bengal, a region in the north of India, was probably reminded of Mount Everest, the peak which had defied all attempts to conquer it until the heroics of Nepal's Sherpa Tenzing and the New Zealander Edmund Hillary on May 29, 1953. Mukherjee conferred on insulin the ultimate title of an insurmountable hurdle by calling it the *Everest of molecules.*

Against the vociferous objections of Swanson, the scientists embarked on the project to create a smaller, simpler molecule just as Hodgkin had done.

(Just how much attention was paid to Robert Swanson, by the scientists, many of whom were already "stars" in the scientific world, is unclear. What is obvious, however, is that Swanson was firstly, younger than most of the scientists involved in the project - he was in his 20s and secondly, Swanson was not known for being backward in coming forward!

It is highly unlikely that he would have had a hope of understanding molecular chemistry even though he had, at least potentially, an expert teacher in Herb Boyer. Swanson had only one goal which was to succeed commercially. Genentech and for that matter insulin were simply a means to an end namely, money.

There were good-humoured comments on Swanson's short stature with a joke in Sally Hughes' *Genentech* that Bob Swanson only looked tall when he stood on his wallet !

The City of Hope scientists led by Itakura, chose *Somatostatin,* a hormone with little market potential but which, like insulin, is produced in the pancreas. However unlike insulin which has 51 amino acids spread over two chains, Somatostatin is a much smaller molecule made up of only 14 amino acids.

Even then Itakura's first attempt at synthesising Somatostatin had failed.

Swanson, who had gathered with the scientists – no one could have kept him out anyway – to watch the much anticipated synthetic, somatostatin was devastated at the failure. He developed severe chest pain and had to be taken to a nearby hospital, emergency unit with a suspected heart attack which, fortunately, turned out to be an attack of severe indigestion.

Undeterred by their first failure Itakura, the molecular chemist known for his tenacity and capacity for spending long hours in the laboratory, was not discouraged. He persisted and, in August 1977, succeeded in producing somatostatin in a test tube.

Under normal circumstances this was a groundbreaking discovery would deservedly call for celebrations, perhaps even self-congratulations, but for the team of Itakura, Riggs, Boyer and Swanson – especially Swanson – the Somatostatin project was but a dress rehearsal. The main goal, and as far as Swanson was concerned, the only goal was insulin.

By the very next morning, the group of scientists and formulated a plan which, was to "attack" insulin, the same verb which had been employed by John Jacob Abel more than 50 years earlier in his letter to Noyes who had persuaded the scientist to look at the newly discovered hormone by Banting and Best in Toronto.

To the modern laboratory warriors, the highly qualified and talented molecular scientists, the project to find the exact structure of the basic unit, the molecule of insulin was more than a contest. It was a battle.

And they were ready to attack.

Insulin in human beings exists as two chains called the A and B chains which are joined with a connecting chain. Separately, neither chain has any effect. Insulin in human beings exists only in the two-chain form.

Recombinant insulin is made by programming bacteria into making the A and B chains.

Each chain is made separately. Then the two chains are joined in the laboratory to produce the insulin in the form it is made in humans who do not have diabetes.

The sequence of steps described above is referred to as *genetic engineering*.

David Goeddel (1951–).

"No one competes with David Goeddel"

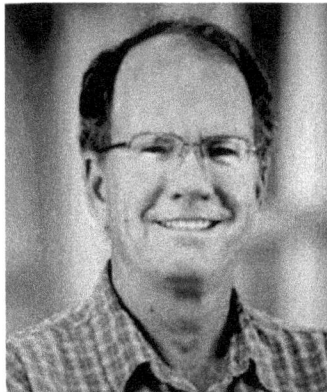

Dave Goeddel.

David Goeddel, was the multitalented 27- year old rock-climber and respected researcher who near midnight, or in the early hours of August 21, 1978 had made history by joining the two chains of insulin. The insulin had not come from the pancreas of an animal. This insulin had been made by bacteria through the experiments carried out by the combined efforts of the team of scientists from Genentech and City of Hope laboratories.

This was the modern insulin.

Goeddel was a strapping, 27-year-old who had been working in Boulder, Colorado when he was contacted to join the team engaged in the insulin project in California.

By his own admission, Goeddel's priorities were rock climbing first, and work, second. In fact he had come to California from Boulder which he had also chosen as a place for his undergraduate studies because its mountain scapes presented challenges in rock climbing.

Why then was Goeddel one of, if not the first scientist to be hired by Swanson and Boyer, the founders of Genentech?

The answer to this question lies in Genentech's first attempt to hire an employee. That employee was not Goeddel but Dennis Kleid, an experienced researcher who was known to Boyer. The two founders of Genentech were delighted when Kleid accepted but were surprised by his insistence that he would not come unless a young researcher in his laboratory was also hired. The young scientist was David Goeddel.

What Kleid had noticed when working with Goeddel was that young man had something that was even stronger than his love of rock climbing. It was his work ethic. On his own admission, Goeddel said that he always wanted "to get it done as fast as possible. And before anyone else". His capacity for hard work was legendary, as was his single-mindedness. In an interview with one of Goeddel's classmates Dan Yansura, Sally Smith Hughes asked if the scientist had worked as rapidly as the rock climber. "No one competes with David Goeddel" was the reply.

Remember, Goeddel was still in his 20s.

After exhaustive, long hours without sleep, the team of young scientists at Genentech, who had had a last-minute hitch with part of the insulin (B) chain, had handed the final back-breaking task to the "ace" researcher David Goeddel, the rock climber with a work ethic which was not for the faint-hearted. His task was to of join the two chains of insulin (called A and B).

Dave Goeddel made history when, deep in the night or the early hours of August 21, 1978 he made the first molecule of modern insulin.

65

MODERN INSULIN DELIVERED

It is useful at this point to recapitulate the steps which culminated in the production of modern insulin.

Paul Berg and his team had produced the first recombinant product (molecule) in the laboratory by combining a piece of DNA, from Escherichia coli, a bacterium, which is plentiful in the intestines of human beings, with a piece of DNA from a simian virus called SV40. The natural host of SV 40 is the monkey.

The method used to join the two pieces was discovered, and developed by Berg, In the jargon of molecular chemistry it is called "splicing."

The team of Paul Berg and his graduate associates including David Jackson and Robert Simmons published their now classical paper in the October 1972 issue of the PNAS (Proceedings of the National Academy of Sciences), one of the most prestigious research publications in the world.

Two years later Boyer and Cohen joined a frog gene with the gene of bacteria. The significant difference between their work and the pioneering studies of Paul Berg was that Berg had joined two viruses, one from E. coli and the second from a tumour virus called SV 40 (Simian Virus 40). As previously stated E. coli lives in the human gut whereas SV40 inhabits the monkey.

Boyer and Cohen on the other hand, had joined a piece of DNA from a virus to the DNA of a frog. On the evolutionary scale a frog is far more advanced than a virus.

In 1976 Boyer and Swanson launched Genentech, the first bio pharmaceutical company.

Finally, on August 21, 1978, David Goeddel joined the A and B chains of synthetic insulin to make the first recombinant molecule of insulin.

Finally Swanson and Boyer, through Genentech, in conjunction with the long-established pharmaceutical company of Lilly delivered modern insulin.

This was the same company which had been instrumental in bringing the original insulin discovered by Banting and his team in Toronto in 1921 to the men, women, and children suffering from diabetes.

The contract signed between Lilly, and Genentech yielded sales of Humulin in the order of $300 million for Lilly in the first year.

The new way to make insulin revolutionised its pharmaceutical production. Since the genetically changed bacteria can multiply indefinitely, the supply of insulin is similarly unlimited.

To make insulin using bacteria such as *E. Coli* which are widespread in nature has forever freed its production from the dependence on the pancreases of slaughtered animals.

Genentech Dazzles the Stockmarket.

Previously unheard of in the stock market with no previous products or earnings record, Genentech's share price took off within minutes from the base of $35 and rose to $89, the largest gain in stock market record to that point.

Seasoned traders were amazed that a biotechnology product could potentially produce a financial windfall and at the same time offer a product which was superior to the drugs or medications in current usage as was the case with Genentech's recombinant insulin.

Sally Smith Hughes in her thought-provoking book *Genentech* (Chicago University Press 2013), highlights the many competing interests which were the nemesis of at least some of the people involved in the production of the original insulin. Smith illustrates the effect of personality on the growth of scientific ideas through her descriptions of the personalities of some of the individuals who contributed to the formation of the company.

Who would have thought it possible that the first biotechnology company could be the result of a collaboration between a venture capitalist like Robert Swanson with a workaholic researcher and the affable academic, Boyer who had been so taken with the Cambridge duo's pursuit of the double helix that he had given his two pet Siamese cats the Genentech was the first biopharmaceutical company to market insulin which was its first major product.

Today there are more than 200 biopharmaceutical companies and more than 300 biopharmaceutical products have been approved by the American Food and Drug Administration (FDA) and the European Medicine Agency (EMA).

The successful manufacture of recombinant insulin will be remembered as the critical breakthrough which saved millions of lives and was the catalyst for the launch of the global biotechnology industry which is now valued at around $500 billion.

The Wider Uses of Genetic Engineering.

Following the development of genetic engineering pioneered by the scientists described in this book, the technique has been used in the production of many medicines including treatment of cancer as well as in improving the quality of livestock and plants.

Most recently, genetic engineering facilitated the development of vaccines to treat the SARS virus during the COVID-19 epidemic.

I struggled to simplify and describe, without using technical terms, the main steps in the method used to make recombinant insulin through Paul Berg's experiments.

I shared the frustrations of the many scientists involved in the exercise as they tried to do the same when being interviewed by non-scientists such as journalists.

The scientist who became quickly known for his capabilities in explaining recombinant technology in lay terms to individuals, including journalists who had little or no scientific knowledge, was

Herb Boyer. Listening to him on YouTube gives a clear demonstration of his remarkable gift in being able to explain complicated scientific information without resorting to technical terms.

Returning briefly to the story of the discovery and development of crystallography, one is reminded of a similar gift possessed by William Henry Bragg who was also admired for his ability to explain complicated matters in simple language.

In this regard Boyer may well be regarded as the William Henry Bragg of modern insulin. Given Boyer's laid-back approach to life, I think he would draw the line at having Bragg's knighthood attached to his name.

Modern Insulin for the Patient.

The unique nature of the collaboration between business and cutting-edge scientific research required the contribution of many individuals. In addition to the laboratory research, there was the challenge of bringing together many scientists engaged in the different parts of the exercise. This amounted to building a team of individuals who had to work towards a deadline determined by priorities which were very different from those usually followed by molecular chemists. In academia the commonest deadline was to get the work published before being beaten to it by others engaged in the same pursuit. For example, making insulin in a laboratory to end the century-long dependence on animal sources was being pursued by at least two other teams in the US alone. However, the deadline which faced the successful team was "a first" for more than a dozen scientists who contributed to the ultimate success of making recombinant synthetic insulin. The new deadline was almost entirely driven by financial motives. The new taskmaster was a non-medical and non-scientist individual – an entrepreneur. Remember that Swanson had been allowed only ten minutes – and that was by an unusually generous, friendly and tolerant Herbert Boyer. So, before describing the many scientists whose contributions gave us the new insulin let us give Robert Swanson the place in history which he deserves for having fought "tooth and nail" to deliver insulin to the millions of men, women and children around the world who use it every day.

Recombinant insulin was promptly utilised in the treatment of patients with diabetes, as soon as it was approved by the Food and Drug Administration (FDA) in 1982. The applicant, Eli Lilly pharmaceutical company promptly launched, and vigorously marketed modern insulin with the brand name *Humulin*.

In retrospect the story of Genentech, the first biotechnology company, is a fascinating account of modern day's young men and women who glimpsed, in a flash of insight a chance for glory, identified and faced up to the challenges, then doggedly stayed the course, went for broke, and against the odds, won.

In doing so they achieved what had been thought unachievable.

66

THE NOBEL PRIZE FOR MODERN INSULIN?

Earlier in this account there was a discussion on the "priority rule" in scientific publications. When it comes to ascribing priority in the formation of a commercial company however, the task is easier.

Although the idea of making, then marketing insulin manufactured through the recombinant technique had been thought of by Herbert Boyer, he had not done anything about it.

It was another young man, an aspiring entrepreneur in his 20s who, with little knowledge of the scientific aspects of recombinant technology, had a "gut feeling" that recombinant technology could be used to market a commercially successful product. His name was Robert Swanson.

Unlike the furore over Banting getting the Nobel Prize for discovering insulin, there was no argument when the award to Paul Berg for pioneering the recombinant technique was announced

By an ironic coincidence, on the day of the public announcement of the launch of Genentech, the first commercial enterprise to market a recombinant biopharmaceutical, an announcement from Stockholm broke the news of the Nobel Prize for Chemistry to Paul Berg. The award was shared withWalter Gilbert and Frederick Sanger for their work on DNA and protein sequencing.

There were many who felt that the actual delivery of recombinant insulin through the critical experiments conducted by Boyer and

Cohen would also have been recognised as being worthy of the "ultimate accolade". Cohen was said to be "nonplussed". Boyer, on the other hand, was philosophical about it, and in an interview expressed his gratitude for what he had achieved as well as his accomplishments in other areas of his life together with the long years of his happy marriage.

That Swanson died in 1999 at the age of 52 is a tragic chapter in the story of modern insulin.

67

PANDEMICS AN ELUSIVE GOAL FOR ANCIENT AND MODERN SOCIETIES

The COVID-19 Pandemic.

"...one of the greatest threats to human health in modern times."

Spokesman, Nobel Committee, 2023.

"... The world had undergone a momentous transformation. Notions of life and death were forever altered. A shadow had fallen and has remained here with us ever since, affecting all sorts of human enterprises, perhaps the greatest of which is the imagination...... and the contagion was quickly spreading. No one knew its cause, and no remedy had proven to have any effect.""

Hisham Matar on the Black Death of 1348.

When COVID-19 descended upon China in 2019, I was working on the biography of Elliott Proctor Joslin, the American pioneer of the treatment of diabetes before the discovery of insulin. I thought the Covid infection would not interfere with my program.

Within days, I realised that I was wrong and subsequent events only served to hammer home this fact. I could not write about the pandemic of diabetes, without addressing the COVID-19 pandemic which remains, still, the issue *du jour.*

The recent world-wide spread of coronavirus, which started as an epidemic in China and rapidly became a pandemic, is fresh in the minds of all. Human history has recorded epidemics from prehistoric times. The "black death" (1346–1353) has been described in journals, books and novels.

One of the most memorable descriptions of the Black Death was by the Tunisian historian Ibn Khaldun, whose work on sociology was described by the English historian Arnold J. Toynbee as "the greatest work of its kind that has ever been created by any mind in any time or place."

Khaldun's whole life was affected by the plague which he had experienced in his childhood at the age of seven. He believed that the major impact of the pandemic had been on human society as a whole:

> *"Civilisation, both in the east, and the west, was visited by a destructive plague, that devastated nations, and caused populations to vanish. It swallowed them up... and wiped them out. Civilisation decreased with a decrease of mankind. Cities and buildings were laid waste, roads and way signs were obliterated, settlement and mansions became empty, and dynasties and tribes grew weak.*
> *The entire inhabited world changed."*

In May 2023, the publishers Simon and Schuster released *Foreign Bodies,* the latest book by the British historian Sir Simon Schama. It recounts various aspects of society's response to pandemics going back to the 14th century's Black Death which afflicted Western Europe, Asia and Africa from 1346 to 1353. The plague is still considered the most devastating infectious disease, killing between 75 to 200 million people.

More recent infections include the Spanish flu of 1918 which ravaged civilian and military personnel during the First World War.

Methods to contain, control or cure the offending infection have met with limited success. For example, smallpox has probably been in existence for several thousand years. Marks on the face of the mummy of pharaoh Ramses the Fifth are said to resemble smallpox, placing the existence of this condition at least 3000 years. Its descriptions are also found in the literature of the Chinese in the fourth, and of India in the seventh century CE (Current Era).

The Covid Pandemic, 2019 and The Story of a Lady in Shanghai.

The COVID-19 Pandemic will go down in history as the modern pandemic and cannot be ignored in any story dealing with current history.

There is still an element of disbelief in any reflection on this deadly affliction, which brought the entire universe to a standstill. Some would say it brought us all to our knees. After all the scientific progress in so many areas ranging from space technology to medical advances had brought most, if not all of us to subscribe to "the sky is the limit" mindset.

In 2003 SARS (Severe Acute Respiratory Syndrome) descended upon and swept the entire world. Starting in China, it quickly engulfed the Americas. Of the initial figure of 8000 people who had caught the virus, nearly 10% perished. A new organism, a new strain of coronavirus was identified as the responsible agent.

On 31 December 2019, a Municipal Health Commission from a city called Wuhan, which previously had not been heard of outside China, reported cases of pneumonia in a small group of people in Wuhan, a city with a population of more than eleven million which is situated at the confluence of the Yangtze and Han rivers, 325 km west of Shanghai.

In January 2020, a business woman in Shanghai had met a 33-year-old German from Munich. Neither had any symptoms of any kind. Shortly, afterwards, the man developed symptoms of the flu. He had returned home and, shortly afterwards had felt well enough to resume work. Nothing more came of it because it was no different from a simple bout of flu, from which most of those who contract the condition recover without complications.

Then, the first hiccup.

The woman in Shanghai, who had been quite well when she had met her German business contact, developed flu-like symptoms and tested positive for SARS-COV2.

To complicate matters further, the man from Munich having recovered completely, when tested was found to have the infectious virus in his sputum.

It quickly became clear that even people without symptoms could carry and spread the highly infectious virus. to make matters worse, the virus also proved to be highly lethal.

It did not take long for Covid to spread right round the world.

Individual experiences and stories spread like wildfire.

Everything stopped.

Lockdown acquired its own connotations, limitations and practices for individuals, for families, for towns and cities, for countries and continents.

From the medical and scientific viewpoint, there were many questions which could not be answered.

One aspect of the response to the Covid pandemic was the rapidity of identifying the organism, causing the infection, and more importantly, developing vaccines to limit its spread. Research went into overdrive and vaccines were developed in several laboratories around the world.

The World Health Organisation (WHO) quickly recognised the potential for the entire world to be affected and issued a series of recommendations for control and prevention.

One of the first cities to be affected by SARS was Hong Kong. The rapid progress of the virus and the large numbers of people affected were alarming. Lessons from the experience in Hong Kong were quickly learned, and this enabled national and international communities to implement effective methods in an attempt to control the spread of the virus.

An early lesson learned from the Hong Kong outbreak was the usefulness of frequent updates of the numbers affected. Daily announcements by leaders of state and nations became the norm in the nightly news telecasts. The importance of isolating the afflicted through home quarantine was recognised and quickly extended to national and international efforts to limit SARS transmission.

The world lived separately – in isolation. Members of the same family living in different suburbs within a large city were separated if they were beyond the limits imposed by local authorities. Short visits to friends or relatives from other countries became prolonged stays. We all feared contact with anyone including family members. Wearing masks was also compulsory – we didn't want to be within range of anyone's breath.

The smallest drop of saliva or mucus from the nose had the potential to infect anyone within range.

Special centres were established where is state-run clinics treated patients with Covid. Telephoning the local general practice to which individuals had been attached, at times for many years, received a recorded message saying, "this practice does not provide treatment for Covid. If you have a cough, cold or fever, or a history of contact with a known case of Covid, you are advised to contact the nearest centre providing treatment."

Governments limited international travel. The care provided for those infected with the virus was compromised because of precautions taken to protect the healthcare providers including doctors, nurses, and allied health professionals. Masks became mandatory. Even the medical profession changed it age-old practice of "physical examination." Doctors, no longer touched patients, and some even stopped using the stethoscopes to listen to the heart or the chest.

International borders were closed. There was cooperation between international bodies, including the World Health Organisation which provided leadership and worked with national bodies such as the US Centre for Disease Control and Prevention (CDC).

A regular feature of the international nightly news saw reports from the US Head of the Centre for Disease Control (CDC), the diminutive Dr Anthony Fauci, who was promptly labelled the "Pandemic Prince" by some newsman.

They emphasised that the pandemic had "caused significant loss of human life and extraordinary disruption."

Lessons learned also acknowledged, at the same time, that "the outbreak continues to change, with new waves of disease affecting different regions of the world and with the appearance of new viral variants" noting the role and importance of widespread vaccination to control COVID-19.

The lockdown employed in most countries to limit the spread of COVID-19 reflects the knowledge gained from the history of global spread of smallpox through the expanding trade routes in centuries gone by. For example, Japan's trade with China in the sixth century had brought smallpox to Japan while Arab expansion led to the infection spreading to northern Africa, Spain, and Portugal. In the 11th century, the Crusaders spread smallpox in Europe and in the 17th century European settlers took that infection to North America. British explorers brought smallpox to Australia in the 18 century.

The success of vaccination is a landmark in the history of smallpox, because in 1980 the World Health Assembly declared the smallpox had been eradicated.

In Australia, State Premiers stood with medical authorities who reinforced medical advice and provided numbers of the newly afflicted, as well as those who had succumbed. The vulnerability of the aged was highlighted by the numbers of the older members of the community who were amongst the dead in the daily count.

Businesses closed.

Schools shut down.

Online activity became an even greater part of daily living and working. Conventional workwear gave way to casual/athletic garments, which in many cases have continued despite the disapproval of some employers.

Educational facilities, including universities, technical colleges, and schools provided information and instruction online.

The fatalities from Covid 19 as of December 2023 number in the order of 6,000,000+.

A Young Doctor's Personal Experience of Covid in Sydney, Australia.

Bill, (real name withheld). the young general practitioner who has provided medical care marked by compassion and kindness to my wife and me in my retirement, was an early victim of Covid which he had caught from a patient.

Previously, he had been an extremely fit individual and a regular cyclist. In addition to usual respiratory symptomsBill developed some of the known complications of Covid in the brain and in the heart. With no history of epilepsy he suffered a seizure. Fortunately he responded to the emergency measures which controlled the fit and he was placed on preventive medication.

But worse was to follow.

As with his seizure, there was no history of any heart problems. So understandably, he was alarmed when he developed a change in his heart rhythm. This also required further urgent treatment.

Bill couldn't work, nor drive because his driver's license had been cancelled after the seizure. The time off work understandably caused apprehension and fear for him and his young family. After several weeks, his condition improved, and fortunately he was able to return to work.

The use of genetic engineering played a crucial role in the rapid development of a vaccine. However, the cost understandably, was substantial. In countries where healthcare was subsidised by the government, the vaccine was available to the elderly, but others had to pay amounts in excess of $1000 for each course of treatment.

When "lockdown" in our state was relaxed and we had been vaccinated, my wife and I wanted to visit our son in Europe. Bill insisted that we buy the vaccine.

"If you have any symptoms, take the treatment," he said. "Don't wait."

As predicted, one of us did develop symptoms of a respiratory infection during our stay in Paris. The vaccine proved to be effective with prompt relief from all symptoms.

It was no surprise that the Nobel Committee recognised the importance of the scientific advances made in the treatment of coronavirus infections and awarded the prize for Physiology or Medicine to two scientists for their studies in mRNA technology and COVID-19 vaccines.

The 2023 Nobel Prize for Medicine and Physiology.

> *"Nothing distracts me from my work."*
> Drew Weissman, Nobel Laureate,2023.

Exactly 100 years after Frederick Banting had won the Nobel Prize for the discovery of insulin, the 2023 Nobel Prize in Physiology or Medicine was awarded to Drs. Katalin Kariko and Drew Weissman. The discovery of insulin by Banting was, in the opinion of most people, deserved to be recognised with the award.

It is worth noting that Drs. Kariko and Weissman had used genetic engineering techniques pioneered by Paul Berg whose scientific accomplishment had played a critical role in the development of modern insulin.

Dr. Kariko, born in Hungary in 1955, is a biochemist best known for her studies in mRNA technology and COVID-19 vaccines. Weissman and Kariko, had carried out their studies at the University of Pennsylvania.

In the words of the Nobel Committee spokesman, the award was given to the two Laureates for discoveries "critical for developing effective mRNA vaccines against Covid 19" during the pandemic that began in early 2020.

The spokesman went on to say that Kariko's and Weissman's work "through their groundbreaking findings, which have fundamentally changed our understanding of how mRNA interacts with our immune system, had contributed to the unprecedented rate of vaccine development during one of the greatest threats to human health in modern times."

Weissman was born in 1959 in Lexington, Massachusetts, and received his MD and PhD degrees from Boston University.

He received his clinical training at Beth Israel Deaconess Medical Centre affiliated with Harvard Medical School.

The Deaconess which was originally the New England Deaconess Hospital, had been established by a body of religious nurses in 1896, has a long association with the history of the study and treatment of diabetes which began with Elliott Joslin, the founder of the Joslin Diabetic Clinic. Joslin was the first Chief Physician of the New England Deaconess Hospital. The establishment of the first dedicated clinic for the ambulatory treatment of patients with diabetes was also established jointly by the Joslin Clinic and the Deaconess Hospital.

68

THE DIABETES PANDEMIC UPSTAGED – AGAIN!

"Don't sleep poet, don't sleep
Do not give into sleep.
You are eternity's hostage
A captive of time.

Boris Pasternak.

"We have the biggest epidemic in the world, and we don't know how to treat it".

Professor David Nathan, Massachusetts,
General Hospital.

As described earlier, epidemics and pandemics of infectious disease such as the plague and tuberculosis have dominated public consciousness when they afflicted mankind over several centuries.

Yet the dramatic increase which has occurred in the number of patients with Type 2 diabetes and is justifiably considered *a pandemic,* fails to make the headlines.

The World Health Organisation's figures for adults (20–79 years) suffering from diabetes in 2021 was in the order of 537 million. It was predicted to rise to 643,000,000 in the following 10 years. The dramatic increase which has occurred in the number of patients with Type 2 diabetes is justifiably considered a *pandemic.*

In the euphoria of acquiring the gift of insulin, Banting could not wait to get the treatment to patients. Some years later an American poet Ogden Nash said,

The pity about a kitten's that,
One day, it'll be a cat.

When one looks back on the discovery of insulin in 1921 and the euphoria which followed the dramatic accounts of the countless lives saved by it, there can be no denying its value in the treatment of diabetes.

Thousands, even millions of patients with Type 1 diabetes around the world were saved.

Before the discovery of insulin, the children and young people with diabetes had an average lifespan of less than five years. Many perished in the first 2 to 3 years, as was the experience of the Boston physician Elliott Joslin, one of the first doctors to establish a clinic exclusively for the treatment of diabetes.

The plight of those who suffered from diabetes before the discovery of insulin was described bluntly but accurately by Walter Campbell, who was the senior physician at Toronto General Hospital at the time of the discovery of insulin in Toronto. Campbell's junior house-officer had given the first injection of Banting's insulin extract to the first human being in that memorable summer of 1922. His comment also referred to adult onset Type 2 diabetes.

Campbell said,

> *"Before the First World War, there were only two types of diabetics, those who died quickly and those who stuck around deteriorating for a long time."*

This was an accurate description of the fate of patients with Type One and Type Two diabetes before the discovery of insulin. "… those who stuck around deteriorating for a long time" refers, one assumes, to Type 2 diabetes.

Insulin has given countless individuals normal lives. They have experienced the joy of accomplishments achieved through training and study. The satisfaction of having families, previously unimaginable, became a reality. Before the discovery of insulin many young people lost their lives by contracting even minor infections such as influenza. With insulin, thousands of young people, some as young as two or three years, recovered from previously fatal infections, and reached adulthood to marry, have children and also pursue careers.

However, the fact remains that the treatment with insulin has now made diabetes a *chronic* condition.

In Frederick Banting's acceptance speech for the Nobel Prize there was not a single mention of the chronic conditions/complications which occur in those whose diabetes has been present for many years. this is understandable since the chronic complications of diabetes only appear several years after the onset of the condition.

It is sobering to recall that gangrene had been recognised in patients with diabetes several hundred years earlier by Avicenna (ca.970–1037), the eminent physician and philosopher of the Islamic world. However it had not been recognised that there was a connection between the duration of untreated or inadequately managed diabetes and the development of conditions such as gangrene. These "complications" are largely due to damage to the blood vessels in different parts of the body. Blockage of the larger arteries in the lower limbs causes gangrene, in the arteries of the heart, angina, heart attacks and heart failure.

The uncomfortable fact is that Type 2 diabetes, although known from prehistoric times, remains undefeated and in the recent years has been described as a pandemic because the number of individuals affected has steadily increased and has now reached alarming numbers. Furthermore, the numbers continue to rise throughout the world and now include the so-called Third World countries.

When the trend was first recognised, affluence was believed to be responsible as an important cause but in the last two to three decades diabetes has spread to affect all sections of communities in nearly every country.

In early 2016, Professor David Nathan, Professor of Medicine at Harvard Medical School and Director of the General Clinical Research Centre and the Diabetes Centre at Massachusetts General Hospital made a statement which would have rung alarm bells for not only his medical audience, but for anyone interested in diabetes. He said, "we have the biggest epidemic in the world and we don't know how to treat it."

Professor Nathan pointed out that at that time (2016), 30 million Americans and 350 million people worldwide suffered from diabetes. He then provided a succinct account of the developments which had followed the discovery of insulin.

Acknowledging that the introduction of insulin in the early 1920s, and given by injection or other devices had been "a major breakthrough" he described the sobering reality of other illnesses which are now seen to accompany (as complications) in those afflicted with diabetes.

Nathan acknowledged that the use of insulin had reduced the rate of blindness in patients with diabetes from 30% to 1%. He also emphasised that whereas in the pre-insulin era kidney failure had afflicted one in five patients and gangrene in feet and legs was a source of indescribable anguish in 12%, treatment with insulin had reduced kidney failure as well as gangrene to 1%.

What is of even greater concern is the admission by medical authorities that none of the strategies employed so far, including education and new drugs, has achieved significant success in slowing, let alone stopping the tide of the rising numbers of men and women developing diabetes.

The alarming increase, especially in adults is now recognised as a major challenge not only for those suffering from diabetes, but also for the providers of health care.

Nationalised health services have had to assign increasing expenditure on diabetes research. The intersection between science and politics has challenged the stakeholders in both fields, especially when it comes to funding research. It would be fair to say that, as a rule, scientists and politicians have little common.

In this book I have written about the role of bureaucrats and administrators such as Flexner's role in Israel Kleiner's research at the Rockefeller Institute and Duncan Graham's treatment of Frederick Banting in Toronto during the initial trials of the insulin extract.

Many of the changes and advances in the knowledge and understanding of diabetes, especially its complications have come from research funded by governments in order to find ways to lighten the burden of the expenditure incurred by the treatment of the complications of diabetes such as loss of lower limbs, heart, failure, and kidney failure.

As a result of such policies, intensive studies have been carried out to further the understanding of the complications of diabetes in the hope of developing more effective treatments. The cost of the treatment as well as the loss from the labour force of individuals afflicted with complications of diabetes has been an important factor in assigning priorities in funding of research by governments and other organisations.

An Early Reminder Unheeded.

In his brief and succinct biography of Elliott Proctor Joslin, one of the early diabetes specialists of the 20th century, the late Donald Barnett wrote of Joslin's comment on the increased incidence of diabetes in the 1920s, fully 100 years before the current awareness of the alarming increase in the numbers, especially in the adult populations of most countries in the world.

Joslin, known, for his clinical acumen, was quoted by Barnett as follows:

> "Although six of the seven persons, all heads of families… living in (three) adjoining houses on a peaceful, elm-lined street in a country town in New England… succumbed to diabetes… no one spoke of an epidemic. Consider the measure which would have been adopted to discover the source of the

outbreak to prevent a recurrence… (as it would)… if these deaths had occurred from Scarlet fever, typhoid fever, or tuberculosis. *Because the disease was diabetes*, and because the deaths occurred over a considerable interval of time, the fatalities past unnoticed."

Elliott P. Joslin, 1921

Early efforts in epidemiology were largely restricted to obtaining information on the number of individuals with diabetes in a given area, namely its incidence.

One such study was conducted by H.L.C. Wilkerson and L.P. Krall in the town of Oxford in Massachusetts in 1947. Krall was a member of Joslin's staff in the Joslin Clinic, which was devoted to the treatment and study of diabetes. Blood and urine tests for glucose identified 4% of the population of 4,983 individuals in the town as having diabetes.

However in recent times studies of the epidemiology of diabetes have been driven largely by the funding bodies including government agencies due to the alarming increase in the cost of treating patients with complications of the disorder.

In Australia, a study in 1980 found that 2.4% of the population was obese. 20 years later, the prevalence of obesity had almost tripled from 2.4 to 7.2%. The causes of this alarming increase were attributed to changes in lifestyle, inactivity, ageing, and for want of a better term, "modernisation" which probably includes several of the factors mentioned above.

Some researchers have raised the possibility of *epigenetics* being a factor.

Epigenetics invokes extreme environmental events such as famine possibly causing an alteration in the behaviour of cells (the DNA) of individuals to make them vulnerable to developing certain conditions such as diabetes.

One of the scientists prominent in the modern insulin story was the late Arthur D. Riggs (1940–2022) who wrote a paper on mammalian epigenetics in 1975 which remains one of the most frequently quoted on the subject.

The Shattuck Lectures on Pandemics.

An interesting recognition of the first Russian flu pandemic of 1889–1890 was through the establishment of the Shattuck lectures. These have continued to the present day. Some of them record observations, even warnings, of the risks of pandemics.

The Shattuck lineage can be traced back to William Shattuck (1622–1672), an early puritan settler in Watertown.

George Cheyenne Shattuck (1783–1854), was a Boston physician.

Like many of the heroes in this book including Frederick Banting, and also many of the young scientists in the story of modern insulin especially Herb Boyer and Stan Cohen, George Cheyenne Shattuck had experienced hardship and poverty. His father had died when young George was only 10 years old. He was educated at Dartmouth College and University of Pennsylvania and practised in Boston from 1807 until his death in 1854. He established the Shattuck Professorship of Pathological Anatomy at Harvard Medical School. Shattuck was President of the Massachusetts Medical Society from 1836 to 1840.

The Shattuck lectures were established by a bequest from Shattuck Snr. who died in 1854. The first Shattuck lecture was delivered in 1890 by George Brune Shattuck, a descendent of the donor. His chosen subject was the "Russian Flu" pandemic in the late 19th century.

Topics for these lectures have been dominated by epidemics and pandemics. Almost all have been devoted to epidemics of infectious disease such as influenza, tuberculosis and, in recent years, the newer infections such as Ebola.

The Shattuck Lecture on Covid - 19.

Global afflictions including the recent COVID-19 pandemic remain the topics favoured for the Shattuck lectures.

These lectures provide a useful record of the response by governments, the medical profession and society in general to various pandemics over the past 130+ years.

Predictably, the 2021 Shattuck lecture, the 131st, was delivered by Anthony Fauci and Eric Rubin on *"Covid-19 in 2021 – Lessons learned and Remaining Challenges."*

Fauci and Ruben, in their 2019 Shattuck lecture had posed three questions:
Where is the pandemic heading?
What are the lessons learned? and
What challenges remain?

All three questions could be directed at those attempting to address and control the diabetes pandemic.

The fourth Shattuck lecture in 1893 was delivered by William Osler, the pre-eminent physician in his lifetime. Osler was himself the subject of the 100th Shattuck lecture given by the popular Dr. H. Brownell Wheeler of Worcester, Massachusetts in 1990.

I mention Osler here for two reasons: firstly, because his lecture on "Tuberculous Pleurisy" dealt with a topic other than an epidemic or a pandemic. In this, he did what Elliott Joslin did in the 32nd Shattuck lecture of 1922 which is described below. The second reason applies to this particular work in that just as Dr. Wheeler was assisted in gathering the material on Osler by Dr Faith Wallis, Head Librarian of the Osler Library at McGill University, some of the material on Osler used in this book comes through the kindly assistance of Professor Milton Roxanas, a member of the Board of Curators of the same McGill Library.

Diabetes, the Hidden Pandemic.

The alarming increase in the numbers of men, women and children affected by diabetes, has failed to attract similar international attention in spite of the prominence given to it in medical textbooks and journals.

This was highlighted in a comment published on March 27, 2015 on the USA National Women's Health Network website:

The Great Diabetes Epidemic…". *this very real threat.*"

In the past few months, there have been two deaths from Ebola in the United States, and half a dozen patients with the disease have been transferred from West Africa to specialised US facilities for treatment. Americans are panicking about the US Ebola epidemic, which has evoked a loud call for public health action – and generated efforts focused on prevention and vaccine development.

> *Now compare that response to the lack of public outcry about the 281,400 deaths in 2010 from a different epidemic: diabetes mellitus! That number is about the population of Toledo, Ohio but the nation has not yet truly mobilised to address this very real threat."*

(Italics by author)

The Shattuck Lecture on Diabetes.

Elliott Proctor Joslin, the highly respected Boston physician delivered the 32nd annual Shattuck Lecture on June 13, 1922. It was published in the Boston Medical and Surgical Journal (today's New England Journal of Medicine) a week later on June 22, 1922.

Joslin emphasised the importance of diet in the treatment of diabetes. Insulin had not come into general use at that time.

He did not comment on the incidence of diabetes, which is understandable because at that time, which was before insulin had become generally available to patients in the United States (or anywhere else except Toronto), a diet restricted in sugar and starches (carbohydrates) was the only treatment available. Joslin, being a firm believer in the benefits of a diet restricted in carbohydrates, devoted his lecture to emphasise the importance of strict adherence to the dietary prescription.

The Shattuck lectures however, were most frequently devoted to the control of diseases which threatened large numbers of people not only in United States, but around the world as evidenced by the actions taken during the Ebola virus epidemic in 2013–2014.

In the United States the control of outbreaks of serious disease and epidemics is carried out through the Centre for Disease Control and Prevention, the CDC. Advice and directives during the recent SARS pandemic were directed by the CDC. Its director Dr. Fauci was seeing frequently on the evening news with updates and changes to medical advice which the CDC considered appropriate.

Even though, as described below, the steady rise in the numbers of patients with diabetes and its complications especially of heart disease, kidney failure, and lower limb amputation from gangrene had been evident for several years, it was only in 1994 that Dr. David Satcher, the Head of CDC described that diabetes had reached "epidemic proportions and should be considered a major public health problem."

Yet diabetes would appear to have crept up on the populations of virtually every country in the last decade, almost by stealth. The reasons for this have not been widely discussed, but the urgency of addressing it is beyond question if one looks at the increasing numbers of middle-aged and older individuals who have diabetes and even more alarmingly, are suffering from its complications such as heart disease, strokes, and gangrene of the lower limbs.

Even a cursory glance at the number of men and women with Type Two diabetes and the blurring of traditional margins of the age at which individuals are prone to fall victim to it, leaves little doubt about the urgency of the situation.

An article by Roger Dobson in the British Medical Journal in 2002 predicted, that the number of people with diabetes will increase by 40% in 2023.

69

INSULIN THE MODERN JOURNEY

The story of modern insulin is one of the most remarkable scientific breakthroughs of modern times.

It began with the creation of insulin, previously a mammalian product, by bacteria.

It was the result of a breathtaking example of the aligning of stars in the world of molecular biology which combined several molecular sciences through the efforts of many researchers in different disciplines in several laboratories in the United States and Britain.

A remarkable confluence of scientific developments, including discoveries of new methods and instruments resulted in producing insulin in a test tube.

As for the transition from the animal derived insulin discovered in Toronto to the modern genetically engineered product, there can be no argument that removing the dependence on animal sources has been a remarkable and long overdue advance in the treatment of diabetes.

To say that the development of modern insulin is a story of remarkable, epoch-making leaps in the understanding and production of insulin would be an understatement. It is also a story of individual and collective accomplishments by exceptionally talented, and determined men and women. Their stories have been described in these pages as well as the transformative changes in techniques and methodologies pioneered and developed in the research laboratories of several countries by a group of remarkable, often colourful, individuals. Most of them were young, and therefore it is of interest to look at the guiding hand of older men and women who acted as mentors and guides.

This narrative describing the history of diabetes as a journey covers thousands of years. It started in the mists of antiquity when the condition was believed to be a manifestation of the wrath of the gods and was mediated through noxious vapours.

It speaks of the history of remarkable men who were teachers and laboratory scientists as well as students and observers of history.

Following the discovery of insulin by an inexperienced medical graduate who was untrained in research, the lives of countless millions received a reprieve from an early death.

Insulin's journey culminated in the discovery of remarkable new methods, culminating in the production of insulin in a test tube without resorting to slaughtering animals for the purpose.

Increased understanding of all the different organs involved in the control of the level of glucose in the blood has led to the development of new agents for the treatment of diabetes. Many of these can be taken by mouth. These spare the patient the inconvenience of injections.

Injections themselves have now been replaced in many instances by devices which provide a more convenient and accurate method of measuring the level of sugar in the blood and delivering automatically precise amount of insulin.

Technological advances have seen an unforeseen and unprecedented leap in the knowledge and facilities available for patients with diabetes as well as those involved in the delivery of medical care

However, it would be unfair to present the current picture of diabetes and its treatment as a rose without thorns.

That the numbers of middle-aged and older individuals all around the world who are suffering from Type II (adult onset)

diabetes is increasing at an alarming rate is a challenge for every government and other instrumentalities involved in the delivery or healthcare.

The pandemic of diabetes, which affects the entire world has so far defied, all attempts to rein in the numbers which are increasing daily. Current estimates of patients with Type Two diabetes are in the vicinity of 460 million while Type One diabetes afflicts 8.75 million.

70

JOURNEYS END

Time, like an ever-rolling stream,
Bears all her sons away;
They fly forgotten, as a dream
Dies at the opening day.

Isaac Watts 1674–1748.

Just as I was starting on this work at the beginning of 2023, Paul Berg died on 15th February, a few months short of 97. Hardly a day passed when over the time I have spent researching and writing about the story of insulin in the larger story of diabetes, that Berg's name did not come up in some context. I stopped to reflect on the work of this peerless scientist who has etched his name in the history of modern scientific achievements. The application of his pioneering recombinant technology has gifted modern insulin to the millions who use it daily.

David Baltimore, a friend and a respected scientist and Nobel Laureate, in the obituary he wrote for Berg said, "the world will be harder to understand without his wisdom."

After ending his collaboration with Herb Boyer, Stanley Cohen now aged 89, returned to research and continued his academic association as Professor of Genetics and Medicine at Stanford.

Herb Boyer, 88 continued as vice president of Genentech until he retired in 1991.

Just before his retirement, he and his wife Grace donated $10 million to Yale School of Medicine to establish the Boyer Centre for Molecular Medicine. This was the largest single donation in the history of Yale School of Medicine. Students of medical history may reflect on the history of donations raised by Yale in the early years of its founding as described in *Joslin A Pioneer in Diabetes Care* (2019).

Even in his senior years, Boyer retained an interest in the outdoors and sport. He found a friend and kindred spirit in his younger colleague, David Goeddel who extended Boyer's interest in fishing to travel to the Arctic in pursuit of that hobby. Boyer delighted in recounting the story of his first trip there in search of cold water fish, which resulted in the two scientists sheltering and shivering in an Arctic storm and not getting a single bite on the fishing lines!

The later lives of many of the pioneers of modern insulin were also marked by their generosity, a reminder that they never forgot their roots. A typical example is Boyer.

Boyer's father had left school at the age of 13, because the death of his own father had left the family without the means to support itself. Boyer's father worked on the railways as a brakeman.

The history of poverty is never forgotten. Neither is life-changing guidance provided by those given to altruistic professions. Boyer had been a typical teenager given to sports and other pursuits of young men until according to his own story his football coach impressed on him, the importance of discipline. There one of the priests, Father Joel Lieb at the Saint Benedictine College, where Boyer went after primary school, had inspired in him an interest in genetic research.

In 2007 the Herbert Wayne Boyer School of Natural Sciences, Mathematics and Computer Studies was established of the Saint Vincent's College, in honour of one of, if not the most distinguished of the college's students.

Boyer's tribute to his time at St Vincent's was expressed as, "St Vincent is a place where you come, hang your hat, and make your way."

Now Professor Emeritus of Biochemistry and Biophysics of University of California in San Francisco, Boyer has lived in California since his retirement.

Bob Swanson who was only 29 years old when with Herb Boyer he had founded Genentech in 1976. The event marked the transformation of the biotechnology revolution into an entrepreneurial, entity, an industry.

10 years after it went public, Genentech in 1990 merged with Roche Holdings of Switzerland in a $2.1 billion merger.

After his retirement Swanson continued his involvement in cultural affairs and served as a trustee of the San Francisco Ballet and the Museum of Contemporary Art. He was "coach Bob" in his daughters' winning soccer teams.

Tragically, at the age of 51 Swanson developed a particularly aggressive form of brain brain cancer and died in December 1999, at the age of 52.

It is a cruel irony that both Fred Banting who discovered and delivered mammalian insulin and Bob Swanson, whose drive and relentless pursuit transported modern insulin from the laboratories of molecular scientists to the bedside of patients with diabetes, died in early middle age.

The possibility of using recombinant DNA to develop other proteins for therapeutic use was seized upon by several scientists.

Insulin became the target of various scientific experiments largely because of the dramatic effect it produced in the lives of men, women and children with diabetes who before the discovery of insulin faced certain death within months, or a few years after developing diabetes.

Why?

One potent reason, which was perhaps all that was necessary to convince interested researchers of the necessity for an alternative method to produce a hormone, was that by the mid 1970s the Eli Lilly Company was using the pancreases from 56 million pigs and cattle each year just to satisfy the US insulin market.

Thus 60 years after the discovery of insulin and it's manufacture from the pancreas of pigs and cattle, the process to make the life-saving treatment independent of a supply of animal products underwent the remarkable transition to being made in a laboratory through recombinant technology which has revolutionised the treatment of diabetes.

Insulin's journey from its discovery to its synthesis took 100 years which when viewed from the point of view of history is but a short excursion in the journey of diabetes which began thousands of years ago in the dawn of written history.

Diligence, cutting-edge technology and backbreaking research over long hours, frequently extending into the early hours of the morning, had succeeded in changing insulin from a covert chemical, into an overt hormone. The Joint Effort (p.313) bears repeating.

The unique nature of the collaboration between business and cutting-edge scientific research required the contribution of many individuals. In addition to the laboratory research, there was the challenge of bringing together many scientists engaged in the different parts of the exercise. This amounted to building a team of individuals who had to work towards a deadline determined by priorities which were very different from those usually followed by molecular chemists. In academia the commonest deadline was to get the work published before being beaten to it by others engaged in the same pursuit. For example, making insulin in a laboratory to end the century-long dependence on animal sources was being pursued by at least two other teams in the US alone. However, the deadline which faced the successful team was "a first" for more than a dozen scientists who contributed to the ultimate success of making recombinant synthetic insulin. The new deadline was almost entirely driven by financial motives. The new taskmaster was a non-medical and non-scientist individual – an entrepreneur. Remember that Swanson had been begrudgingly allowed only ten minutes –and that was by an unusually generous, friendly and tolerant Herbert Boyer. So, before describing the many scientists whose contributions gave us the new insulin let us give Robert Swanson the place in history which he deserves for having fought "tooth and nail" to deliver insulin to the millions of men, women and children around the world who use it every day.

Little wonder that insulin has been referred to as "a daily miracle."

As is seen repeatedly in history, the names of the many illustrious men and women who gave of themselves to improve the lot of the suffering maybe forgotten but the fruits of their labours will forever adorn the annals of recorded human experience.

The End

Postscript

Preserving History in the Electronic Age

A valuable resource for this work was the book *Genentech* by Sally Smith Hughes (University of Chicago Press, 2013.) which contained information on the scientists who were prominent in the recombinant insulin story and participated in the formation of the pioneering biotechnology company Genentech.

As I read the impressive work, I was especially drawn to the amount of detail the author provided in her stories of different individuals who were prominent in the pursuit of recombinant insulin. Similarly, the body of information on the formation of Genentech contributed significantly to make her book not only an important addition to the literature on the subject but also an enjoyable reading experience. When I turned to the references at the back of the book, I was surprised to realise that I was reading about events as described by the scientists who were actually involved in the dual roles of creating the new form of insulin as well as engaging in the formation of the biotechnology company.

This led to yet another discovery I made in the course of writing this book. This was the important role of oral history collections.

Oral History Collections, a Brief History.

The History of Medicine Division of the National Library of Medicine, formed by four librarians and four physicians in Philadelphia on May 2nd, 1898 during the reign of Queen Victoria, had begun an oral history initiative in the 1960s.

The spoken word is the ideal medium of information for those who are no longer able to read the written or printed word.

The history of the development of modern insulin through recombinant technology includes an impressive body of material from oral history as related by many of the participants and contributors involved in the project from its inception to the establishment of the early biotechnology companies including Genentech which occupies a central role in the history of modern insulin.

The importance of oral history as a research technique was recognised during the Second World War. subsequently, technological advances, such as sound, recording on magnetic tapes, provided a method of storing speeches, lectures, and interviews. By the 1970s, sound recordings on magnetic tape had become commonplace and cassettes were used as a convenient and relatively safe form of storage.

It was from such a form of storage that Charles Best's Osler oration which had been preserved on a magnetic tape was transcribed by my late secretary Cheryl Fleming for inclusion in *100 Years of Insulin* published on the Centenary of the use of insulin in the treatment of diabetes.

Even though the oral record can include personal impressions, it also provides the listener with the impressions or views of the famous as well as ordinary men and women whose story is recorded as part of history.

Relevant to this work is the collection of recordings on the history of biotechnology which was launched by the Bancroft library, University of California, Berkeley in 1996. The university is located near several biotechnology companies.

In order to preserve the recollections and written papers of university and corporate scientists including the pioneers involved in creating the biotechnology companies, the Bancroft library established a program in1996.

In relation to the research behind the development of modern insulin the age of most of the scientists permitted the writers of articles, and books on the subject to approach the main players directly. It is clear that all these scientists displayed the humility. typical of most accomplished men and women. Without exception they were candid and humble when it came to discussing their findings relating to experiments on insulin.

Genentech made a significant commitment in 2001 to provide the library's program with documents and recordings of recollections by many of the scientists involved in the development of recombinant insulin, as well as in the establishment of Genentech.

The library has built up a collection of research material, including oral history, transcripts, archival collections and personal papers of relevance to the history of biotechnology, not only in academia, but also in industrial settings. The library's advisory board includes prominent individuals in the academic as well as in industrial fields to help in the direction of the oral history and archival components held in this part of the Bancroft library.

The method followed to establish the program has been in use since the founding of the regional oral history office in 1954. It houses some 2000 oral histories. The material includes research in primary and secondary sources as well as recorded interviews and transcripts of most interviews. The transcripts are edited by the interviewer but finally reviewed and approved by the interviewee. Bound volumes of transcripts include table of contents, introduction, interview, history, and index, as well as cataloguing in UC, Berkeley, and National Online Library, on networks, as well as announcements and notices in scientific medical and historical journals, and newsletters.

The online availability of live interviews conducted by Sally Smith Hughes, of some of the individuals involved in developing modern insulin provides a fascinating and valuable chapter in the narrative.

Similarly, the history of establishing Genentech, the first commercial company to market a biotechnological pharmaceutical by taking recombinant insulin out of the laboratory and making it available on the market provides the reader with an insider's view of the drama as it unfolded.

Watching Paul Berg, Herb Boyer, Norman Cohen and David Goeddel speaking was like getting a ringside seat to witness the drama as it had unfolded.

Oral history has also occupied an important role in preserving history in England. The Brotherton Library at the University of Leeds provides access to recordings, such as a conversation between Dorothy Hodgkin and Robert Robinson during which I heard Hodgkin saying, "you had put insulin into my hands in 1935…"

Dorothy Hodgkin had won the Nobel Prize for Chemistry in 1964 for her work on insulin, penicillin and other molecules.

It was stimulating, to say the least, to listen to Dorothy Hodgkin whose work illuminates the discovery and development of insulin as described in this book. She was speaking to the late Sir Robert Robinson, Nobel Laureate and former President of the Royal Society (1945 - 1950).

To actually hear the voice of this remarkable scientist, mother, wife, and peace-activist, some 30 years after her death was an experience which justified all the hours I had spent on writing this book. I cannot think of a greater privilege or a more fitting way to end this story.

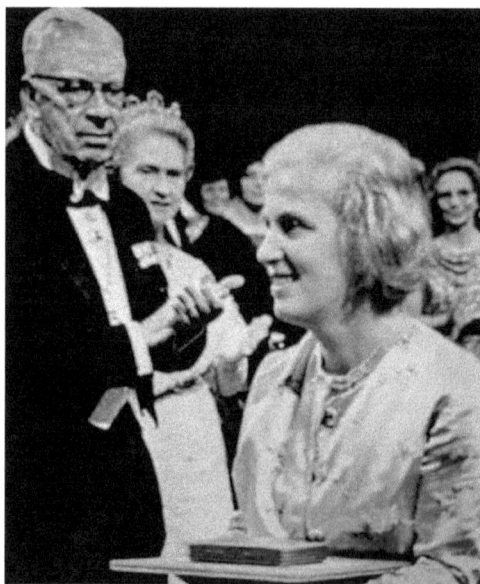

Dorothy Hodgkin (1910-1994).

Historical Chronology
Insulin

A brief historical chronology of modern insulin.
Its creation and commercialisation.

1947: Robert Arthur Swanson is born.

1970: Swanson graduates from M.I.T.

1975: Swanson organises luncheon to interest scientists in commercial production of recombinant insulin – but fails.

1975: Swanson sacked by venture capitalist employers.

1975: Swanson learns that scientists predict 10 to 20 years before recombinant insulin can be produced profitably.

1975: Swanson realises that advising new companies is like being "a coach on the sidelines" and decides to form his own company.

Swanson's cold - calls rejected by all scientists (researching recombinant technology) except Herb Boyer.

1976 (January): Swanson meets Herbert Boyer without knowing of Boyer's expertise. 3 hour pub lunch.

1976 (March): Swanson takes business plan to venture capitalists who, only after meeting Boyer, invest $100,000.

1976 (April 7): Genentech registered with Perkins (head of the venture capital firm) as Chairman, Swanson its President, Boyer the Vice President.

1978: Genentech and City of Hope scientists produce bio- synthetic human insulin using recombinant DNA technology which used E. coli bacteria. This was the Genentech Company's first marketable product.

1980: Genentech raises 35 million through an IPO (initial public offering.

1982: FDA approves human insulin cloning.

1982:Eli Lilly Company having successfully brokered a relationship with Genentech markets Humulin (trade name), the first modern human insulin created in a test tube without depending on animal sources.

Timeline of Biotechnology

Timeline of the Birth of the Biotechnology Industry.

1912: William Henry Bragg develops crystallography.

1925: John Jacob Abel isolates insulin crystals.

1928: Frederick Griffith discovers transformation principle during World War 1(1914–1918). Publishes findings in 1928.

1944: Oswald Avery isolates DNA. Publishes findings in 1944.

1953: Frederick Sanger demonstrates amino acid sequence of insulin.

1960: Rosalyn Yalow describes radioimmunoassay. of insulin.

Early 1968: Paul Berg's sabbatical with Renato Dulbecco. Berg changes his direction of research to virus SV 40.

Winter, 1968: Berg returns to Stanford. Berg continues with the sabbatical studies.

Winter 1970 :Berg works with a team incl. Jackson and Morrow.
:Janet Metz joins Berg's team.
:Metz meets Boyer who facilitates Metz's research.

Late 1970: Berg develops 1st recombinant molecule.

1972: Asilomar: advises caution in recombinant research. The voluntary two year moratorium on recombinant research is not observed by all scientists.

November1972: Boyer and Cohen hatch a plan in Honolulu Deli.

February 1973: VW shuttle service from Cohen's laboratory to Boyer's to jointly pursue recombinant insulin.

New Year's Day 1974: Cohen and Boyer succeed in joining a frog gene with a bacterial gene.

1974: End of Cohen-Boyer Collaboration. Cohen joins Cetus and returns to own research. Boyer returns to his University appointment.

January 1976: Swanson meets Boyer - 3 hour meeting. :Venture capitalists join after Boyer's explanation of recombinant technology.

April 7th, 1976: Genentech launched.

August 1978: David Goeddel of Genentech makes first modern insulin molecule.

October 14th,1980: Genentech announces itself on the stock market.

October 14th,1980: Announcement of Nobel Prize for. recombinant technology to Paul Berg.

28th October1982: Modern insulin, trade name *Humulin,* the first recombinant product for human use made by Genentech is marketed by Lilly.

1983: Humulin, is released on the market for the treatment of diabetes.

Timeline of Banting's Experiments.

October 31, 1920: reads the article by Moses Barron and dreams.

November 1, 1920: approaches Professor Miller, his supervisor for guidance.

November 7, 1920: Banting travels to Toronto for meeting with Professor Macleod.

April 1921: Macleod assigns Charles Best to help Banting.

May 16, 1921: Banting organises the laboratory to start his project.

May 17, 1921: Banting operates on the first dog with Macleod assisting.

July 30, 1921: First effective extract injected in dog number 410.

August 9, 1921: Both researchers report their success to Macleod who is on holidays in Scotland.

August 15, 1921: The experiment which convinced Banting. At midnight Dog 92 was given the extract and dog 409 was not. The next morning Banting discovered that Dog 92 was thriving and the untreated dog, 409, had died.

September 6, 1921: Macleod writes back to caution against premature celebration citing Kleiner's work as being similar.

November 14, 1921: Banting presents results of his experiment add to the Physiology Journal Club of Toronto University. An older professor suggests a "longevity experiment".

November 18, 1921: Longevity experiment started on dog 33, "Marjorie."

December 6, 1921: Marjorie treated with extract for 70 days. Blood sugar remains well controlled.

December 12, 1921: Banting and Best experiment successfully on dog 35 with extract from bovine pancreas.

Mid December 1921: JB Collip joins Banting to improve the quality of the extract.

January 11, 1921: first injection of Banting's extract given to Leonard Thompson failed to benefit the patient.

January 23, 1922: 1st successful injection of Banting's extract to Leonard Thompson.

References

Able, J.J. Crystalline Insulin. Proceedings National Academy of Science. USA 1926, 12, 132–136. (Google Scholar).

Adams, M.J. ; Hodgkin, D.C. et al. Structure of Rhombohedral Zinc Insulin Crystals. Nature 1969, 224, 491–419.

Attie, A.D, Tang, Q Bornfeldt, K.E. The insulin centennial. J Biol. Chem. 2021 Nov; 297.

Butler S.F.B: Two Nobel Laureates in conversation…Notes Rec. published online, 14 July 2021.

Campbell, K.D.: Robert Swanson, 52, alumnus who launched biotechnology industry. MIT News, December 8, 1999.

Chaudhury, A et al: Clinical Review of Antidiabetic Drugs: Implications for Type 2 Diabetes. Frontiers in Endocrinology. Published online.2017.00006.

Cushing, H. The Life of Sir William Osler. Volume Two. Oxford University Press. 1940.

Dobson, R.: BMJ 2008, June 8.: Number of people with diabetes will increase by more than 40% by 2023.

Flier J.S. and Kahn R: Insulin: A pacesetter for the shape of modern biomedical science and the Nobel Prize. Mol. Metabolism 2021 October; 52:101194.

Friedman, J.: World War I And The Fatal Delay In Treating D Diabetes. Harpers, November 2018.

Gale E.: Sir Harold Himsworth. Int. J. Epidemiology: 42, 6. 2016.

Jaskolski, M. Dauter, Z.W. Wlodawer. A brief history of macromolecular crystallography, illustrated by a family tree and its Nobel fruits. The FEBS Journal Vol.281, Issue 18, pp 3985–4009.

Hall, S.S: Invisible Frontiers: The Race to Synthesise a Human Gene. Sedgwick and Jackson, London, 1988.

Jaskolski M. et al.: A brief history of macromolecular crystallography, illustrated by a family tree and its Nobel fruits. FEBS Journal September 2014 pp. 3985–4009.

D.A. Jackson, RH Symons, P. Berg: Biochemical method for inserting new genetic information into DNA of Simian Virus 40. Circular SV40 DNA molecules containing lambda phage genes and the galactose operon of Escherichia coli. Proceedings National Academy Sci. USA, 69, 2904–2909 (1972).

Levene, PA. Studies in Phloridzin glycosuria. Journal of Physiology (1894), 17: 259–71.

D. Lynn Loriaux, MD, PhD. Diabetes and the Ebers Papyrus 1552. Endocrinology, Diabetes, and Clinical Nutrition: 2006, 16, 2, p. 55-56.

Osler Sir William: An Encyclopedia. C.S. Brian Editor. The American Osler Society 2020.

Owens, D.R. Human Insulin: Clinical Pharmacological Studies in Normal Man. Lancaster: Springer Science & Business Media (2012).

Roth J. et al: DIABETES / METABOLISM RESEARCH and REVIEWS, 2012; 28: 293–304.

Roth J. et al. Insulin Discovery: New Insights on its 90th Birthday. Diabetes / Metabolism Research and Reviews, 2012; 28: 293–304.

Scott, D.A. Crystalline Insulin. Biochemistry Journal, 1934, 28, 1592–1602. (Google Scholar).

Stern S.: The Case of Synthetic Insulin. NIH Library of Medicine.

Templer S: MJA 2023: 219 (10) 457- 450.

Vecchio I et al: The Discovery of Insulin: An Important Milestone in the History of Medicine. Front Endocrinology (Lausanne) 2018; 9: 613.

Wright J.R and McIntyre L. Misread and Mistaken: Ettienne Lancereaux…: Journal of Medical Biography. 2022 vol. 30 (1) 15–20.

Zimmet, P and Alberti, G.M.: Diabetes Care. 2016 June: 39 (6): 878–883

Zinman B, Skyler J.S et al: Diabetes Research and Care Through. the Ages. Diabetes Care 2017, 40: 1302–1313.

Nobel Lectures : F.G. Banting P. Berg, J. Macleod, R. Yalow. Oral History & Interviews: Hodgkin and Robinson, Charles Best, Stanley Cohen, Dan Yansura, Herb Boyer Videos & UTube: P. Berg, D. Goeddel, S.N. Cohen, H. Boyer, H.W. Bragg, Dave Goeddel, Joslin Archives: John Brooks CEO, Matt Brown Archivist, Dr. D.M. Barnett and Dr. Donna Younger.

Bibliography

Genentech. Sally Smith Hughes (Chicago University Press) 2023.

The Gene. An Intimate History. Siddhartha Mukherjee (Scribner 2016).

Treatment of Diabetes Mellitus. Elliott P. Joslin. 3rd, 13th & 14th Editions.

A Diabetic Manual for the Mutual Use of Doctor and Patient. EP, Joslin, Lea and Febiger. Philadelphia, 1937.

Margaret and Charlie. Henry Best.

The Discovery of Insulin. Michael Bliss.

Elliot P Joslin : A Centennial Portrait. Donald M. Barnett.

A Month in Siena : Hisham Matar. Penguin Books, 2020.

Sir William Osler: An Encyclopedia. Editor Charles S.Bryan.

The Life of Sir William Osler Volume 1. H. Cushing. Oxford University Press 1940.

The Immeasurable World. A Desert Journey. Atkins, W. Faber and Faber, 1988.

Say Nothing. Patrick Radden Keefe. William Collins, 2018.

100 Years Of Insulin. S K Sinha (online publication) 2022.

Joslin A Pioneer in Diabetes Care. S.K. Sinha, (online publication) 2019.

Acknowledgements

Many physicians and scientists have made important contributions to the knowledge of diabetes and insulin which are the subjects of this work. Though not referenced individually, this work remembers them. The use of online references to check on isolated facts such as dates of birth and death and family details through search engines including publications from the National Institute of Health, Google and Wikipedia made my task much easier and their assistance is gratefully acknowledged.

Vijendra Kumar, a childhood friend since we were 13-year-olds in a boarding school remains a friend and guide.

Throughout the time devoted to this work I have been given willing and enthusiastic assistance from many colleague and friends including Professor Munichoodappa "Muni", from Bangaluru, India for sharing not only the clinical details of how diabetes has affected him, but also how it has affected several members of his family. Muni, whom I have known for more than 50 years, has been a friend from the time of our Fellowship at the Joslin Clinic in Boston in the late 1960s and has helped me during my preparations for writing books on diabetes for the lay public.

Professor Suresh Mehtalia provided me with information on the late Dr Rachmiel Levine with whom he had worked in New York in the late 1960s.

Professor Eberhard Standl of Munich, Germany is another Joslin associate who, like Muni, has written books on diabetes. Eberhard has been ever willing to provide information and advice on this and my earlier wrtings. I was also appreciative of his willingness to provide details of his father's and grandfather's impressive medical accomplishments. Eberhard agreed to let me write about his athletic accomplishments which was a pleasure and a privilege.

Georges Lentz provided willing and helpful assistance with translations from French and German to English.

Professor Jeffrey Friedman from the Rockefeller Institute New York, USA graciously allowed me to draw on his article *Discovery Interrupted* in Harper's magazine, November 2018.

Anna Fienberg, a much loved author of children's books, provided information on her father the late Dr. Len Fienberg as did Professor James P. Isbister on his father Dr.James Isbister Snr. who was my friend and mentor.

Professor Milton Roxanas, is a close friend who shares my interest in medical history. Milton, Ernest (Dr.Ernest Tam, Head of Geriatrics at Ryde Hospital), and I discuss topics of common interest during our regular lunchtime meetings. Milton has provided several references used in this book. Much of the information on William Osler also comes from Milton who is a member of the American Osler Society and a member of the Board of Curators of the Osler Library in McGill University, Canada.

My younger colleague and Medical advisor who remains unnamed for ethical reasons, is featured in the section on Covid.

Michael Lockwood, a friend for many years and an expert on photography has provided advice and assistance with photographs and scanned images.

Professor Paul Fishburn helped with photographs for the cover the book.

Isabel Redden, a retired librarian, provided willing and helpful advice on various aspects of presenting this work.

Andrew Burgess provided feedback from a general reader's perspective.

Warren Reed, a respected novelist, has been a friend and guide from the beginning of my journey in writing.

Tilak Sinha provided the digital image which was the subject of the painting used on the cover.

Our grandson Sean was unfailing in his willing and prompt answers to my word-processing questions.

Every mistake in this book is mine, and I humbly apologise for each one.

Finally, I thank Lee for her many practical suggestions, infinite patience and constant support as I spent many hours alone working on this book. Lee's painting of a scene from the village of Meursault in Burgundy is featured on the cover of this book.

Index

www.ingramcontent.com/pod-product-compliance
Lightning Source LLC
Chambersburg PA
CBHW041254040426
42334CB00028BA/3013